oven
facile

Clinical Hypnotherapy: A Transpersonal Approach

(Revised Second Edition)

An Educational Guidebook

by

Dr. Allen Chips

I

Transpersonal Publishing
PO Box 7220, Kill Devil Hills, NC 27948

Orders:
Wholesale—www.TranspersonalPublishing.com
Retail—www.Holistictree.com

First printing, first edition: September, 1999
Second printing, second edition: September, 2004
Third printing, second edition: February, 2006
Fourth printing, revised second edition, October, 2010

ISBN 978-1-929661-08-4 (softcover edition)
ISBN 978-1-929661-09-1 (hardcover edition)

Line Art Illustrations by Allen S. Chips
Sketched Illustrations by K. Dee Chips
Photo Illustrations & Cover Design by Allen S. Chips

Unattributed quotations are by Allen Chips

All Transpersonal Publishing titles, imprints, and distributed lines are available at special quantity discounts for bulk purchases for sales promotions, premiums, fundraising, and educational or institutional use. For details, contact the Publisher through websites or email.
No author queries please.

Printed in the United States of America

Dedication

This book is dedicated to Dee Chips, my wife. With God, she introduced me to this field, and I have had a thirst for knowledge that has stemmed from this work ever since. She has been supportive of my writing and teaching career and is known by many in this field as my counterpart. She is a unique, intelligent, and helpful person to all who cross this path; as one popular writer and trainer in the field described her, "Even if you scratch down to the other layers, you still find good."

Acknowledgments

Much "thanks" goes to Wayne Halyn, Inanna LaFevre, and Marjorie Reynolds for helping us with several of the well-needed edits of the first edition, which led to this revised, second edition; Dee Chips for sketching a number of the illustrations and proofing; Stanley and Jane Chips for parental encouragement to finish the first edition, which took me three years; and the Lexington Coffee Roasting Company Owners Terry & Melissa Scholl for letting me write the bulk of the first edition in the coffee roasting room, which provided well needed aroma therapy.

Contents

Tables and Illustrations

Introduction

How I became interested in hypnosis...

I was introduced to hypnosis in January, 1981, when I was a freshman at West Virginia University. It all began when I met a very nice esoteric girl that I bonded with right away. It was as if we had known each other all of our lives, which was very peculiar for me. I was very traditional in my religious beliefs at that time, but open-minded enough to listen to this very interesting girl's theories of reincarnation. Shortly thereafter, she found a psychology student in graduate school who used hypnosis to conduct past-life regressions. Upon hearing about her discovery of the service, and because I didn't want the hypnotist controlling her mind, (my misperception at the time), I went with her to attend the session.

We met in a small dark conference room in the back of the Mountain Lair, which was the student arts and activities center at West Virginia University. The hypnotist lit a candle and began inducing hypnosis. After some eye fixation exercises, deepening techniques, and the assistance of her guardian angel as her guide, this courageous college freshman began to experience images from another place and time. As she was experiencing the images and describing them to us, I began to actually experience similar images myself. The images, which appeared to be memories of World War II, began to flood my mind like a torrential rainstorm that wouldn't cease. As the story unfolded, I was getting more and more details about the scenes, even before she described them. Her memory went from a special room where her spirit guide led her to view herself as a male medic on an island in the South Pacific who was dedicated to repairing the bodies of both sides. In the next scene, he was coming back from the war to his would-be fiancee and her mother, who were eagerly awaiting his safe arrival. I was particularly affected by her telling of the loss of his sweetheart's brother, who did not return from the war, and I began to empathize deeply. I must have gone into trance at the same time...what I now refer to as "piggy backing," in order to have had what appeared to be a simultaneous regression experience.

I found it highly unusual that I, a devout conservative Christian, would have such an emotionally gut-wrenching experience simply from observing a hypnosis session of a girl who was supposedly nothing more than a warm acquaintance. The images that entered my mind's eye put me on an emotional roller-coaster ride that involved love, loss, and a myriad of realities only experienced by those who had lived through war times. I had always detached myself from World War II history books and conversations throughout my life; yet, at that time, it took all my effort to regain my composure in front of the others during and after that session.

Afterward, I was very reserved while we walked back to our dormitories together, and I had a difficult time expressing what I had experienced. Surprisingly, I found myself filling in a lot of the gaps in the story from another viewpoint. As we easily got to know each other over the next few months, we compared notes on our experiences, and the details of each other's memories were consistent.

Shortly after that experience, I fell in love with this girl, who later became my wife, and we became the proud parents of two children. Over the next several years, I set out to research and experience hypnosis and read everything that I could get my hands on, while I nurtured a rapidly accelerating medical marketing career. Many clinical hypnotherapy books led me into self-hypnosis, past-life therapy, hypnoanesthesia, habit cessation, and more. I then became bored with the corporate fast track and decided that I would make a change.

I became a certified hypnotherapist and opened my first hypnotherapy center. I was soon busy with a wide variety of clientele. I then began working in a psychiatric group setting at the same time. Shortly thereafter, I received a doctorate degree in clinical hypnotherapy and my wife and I began teaching certification programs in hypnotherapy and reiki healing, another holistic healing art.

We teach a wide variety of methods and interventions, and only part of our emphasis is on "abstract regression" as I call it, or what most refer to as "past-life regression therapy." Through years of research into this particular phenomenon, I must say that I am not convinced that all past-life memories are absolutely what they appear to be in every case. There are many possibilities for the source and nature of these memories, which I further discuss in the chapters titled Abstract Regression and the Cayce Effect.

My goal in writing this book is simply to spread the awareness of this unusually powerful healing modality as far as possible. Although this book does not include all of my advanced theories and methodologies, it does take the student of hypnotherapy from foundational concepts to advanced hypnotic regression techniques. From this level, the student is referred to other resources. My hope is that other hypnotherapy trainers will include this text as a reference, or perhaps they will use it as their core training text for students desiring entry-level instruction. In addition, those who have already had formal hypnotherapy training will find this to be a refreshing approach to practicing clinical hypnotherapy. In addition to methods that I have personally developed over almost two decades, I believe this book combines some of the best clinical methods of other writers in the field. Also making this book unique are sound methodologies encased within a well-grounded transpersonal perspective.

Transpersonal may be defined as "the crossing of body,

mind, and spirit." If you believe that we are of a spiritual origin, and that the altered state is the bridge for linking ourselves to our physical and spiritual dimensions, then this is the right book for you. With this perspective in mind, I welcome you to begin the one journey that does not end, the study of *the mind.*

About This Book

Hypnosis generally involves the subjective experiences of hypnotherapists and their clients. Because of this, I will use interchangeable terms to describe the same concepts (hypnosis, altered state, trance, etc.). Though various terminology used will be defined to some degree in each chapter, accessing the glossary and/or index at the back of the book may be beneficial to the reader for further clarification. Also, the text in this book was slightly enlarged for the visually impaired.

Another very important aspect of this writing is how you will be challenged to define your own beliefs regarding the inner components of self that are at work within the altered state of hypnosis. Unlike other writings on the subject of hypnosis, the mind, body, and spirit will be emphasized for the purpose of expanded understandings. There is no other published work that I am aware of at this time that clinically integrates these aspects into the practice of hypnotherapy as this book does. As you take this journey with me, we will hypothesize together over clinical methodologies and their effects on the mind, body, and spiritual dimensions. When I use the word "spirit" in this work, it should be a given that you believe in human beings having a spiritual nature that is present both internally and externally: internally in the theory that we are created in the image of a higher being or force and, in part, contain that force within; and externally in that a higher power, " God" or the "Great Spirit," has the ability to affect our mind and body for a spiritual directional shift, or higher purpose, which can be individually grasped and understood. Metaphorically speaking, I hope to create an effect which appears as if spirit were watching over us from above, smiling, with a unique understanding of the potentiality we have to understand ourselves within the human plight.

With this higher perspective on the work, and considering the awesome power of the mind, we will learn a great deal about our abilities to create change on multiple levels. My hope is that through this approach we find commonalities in this widely subjective and somewhat controversial subject matter. We may question what makes hypnosis such a powerful intervention for change and new awareness, but because we largely theorize to understand it, a wide variety of opinions over this material hold equal weight. In other words, as I often tell those who attend my seminars, "I'm not here to give you answers. I'm here to provide you with tools and stories of my experiences, so that you can come up with your own answers to the hypnotherapeutic experience."

My observations and opinions, like every one else's, are derived from my studies and experiences, even though such experiences involve thousands of individual human minds. It will be up to each of you to turn the *knowledge* you gain from this book into *wisdom* by putting into practice the valuable concepts you learn herein.

My hope is that you may receive my writings as another piece to the puzzle of the human mind, which I believe, with its higher spiritual connectedness, contains the answers to the universe. Considering this probability, I believe the mind is the true *final frontier*. So... as many back packers have been known to say when crossing paths and departing into the wilderness, "Happy trails."

Chapter I

Defining Hypnosis

Hypnosis may be classified as an *altered state of consciousness* (ASC). In most instances the terms "altered state of consciousness" and "hypnosis" can be used synonymously; the reason being, most ASCs must involve what are considered to be traditional hypnotic techniques, and conversely, hypnosis contains many of the same tools that are utilized in other altered states of consciousness.

Altered States of Consciousness

In order to define hypnosis, we must first look at *Normal States of Consciousness (NSC)*, defined by C.T. Tart as the state in which an individual "spends the major part of his waking hours."[1] A. M. Ludwig defines *Altered States of Consciousness* as a "mental state induced by various psychological, physiological or pharmacological maneuvers or agents, which can be recognized subjectively by the individual himself...as representing a sufficient deviation in subjective experience of psychological function from certain general norms for that individual during alert, waking consciousness."[2] My own definition of altered states of consciousness can be summarized as follows: *a shift in a person's consciousness which can be subjectively and/or objectively distinguished from the mental processes that generally exist in the waking state.*

The concept of *Usual Altered States of Consciousness (UASC)* is a term I created to describe "hypnotic or altered states of consciousness in which individuals enter into automatically and involuntarily on a regular basis." Sleeping, day dreaming, and biochemical shifts—such as fevers, psychotropics, or drug usage—are all examples of UASCs.

Another classification that I created to describe altered states of consciousness includes *Applied Altered States of Consciousness AASC*. These may be defined as "hypnotic or altered states of consciousness which we apply to ourselves and others by some combination of mental and physical procedures and which are intended to create specific outcomes." Interestingly, most of the individuals that use *Applied Altered States of Consciousness,* such as meditation, prayer, and creative visualization, are unaware that they are using forms of hypnosis, or ASCs, to enable the outcome which they are attempting to achieve.

For example, the nurse using creative visualization in the oncology department will notice that some of the patients appear to be nodding off. This is because he or she is using hypnosis, and the most susceptible patients are spontaneously entering into the deepest levels. The nurse is unintentionally using hypnosis, without calling it such or intending the deeper somnambulistic result. Most modern-day hypnotherapists use creative visualization, at least in part, as an important component of an effective hypnotic induction, although sometimes it is used alone as the primary hypnotic induction.

All altered states of consciousness can be classified as forms of hypnosis. Hypnosis is an altered state of consciousness, as are all those listed in Table 1-1.

Table 1-1
Classifications of States of Consciousness

State	Classification
Waking	NSC
Strong Emotions	UASC
Daydreaming	UASC
Television	UASC
Dreaming	UASC
Sleeping	UASC
Pharmacological Agents	UASC
Biochemical Shifts	UASC
Hypnogogic	UASC
Meditation	AASC
Biofeedback	AASC
Transcendental Meditation	AASC
Prayer	AASC
Creative Visualization	AASC
Neurolinguistic Programming	AASC
Reiki	AASC
Guided Imagery	AASC
Guided Meditation	AASC
Yoga	AASC
Progressive Relaxation	AASC
Hypnosis	AASC

All of the definitions of the ASCs in the table above can be found in the glossary in the back of the book. The two primary distinguishing factors between each of the altered states of consciousness listed in Table 1-1 involve the *means* used to enter into the altered state and the *experience* which occurs once the state is achieved. In other words, we may define the tools used to enter into an ASC, *and* the purpose of going there, and thereby find the appropriate label for our experience. The primary factor that distinguishes hypnosis from the other AASCs is that hypnosis is a much deeper AASC than any of the others. It is simply a greater in-depth study of how people relax. People are able to enter into an ASC more easily and to a deeper level by using hypnosis techniques.

Generally speaking, hetero-hypnosis (the act of applying hypnosis to another individual), or hypnotherapy, is more likely to facilitate the achieving of a deeper altered state than the majority of its neighboring ASCs (more of the reasons for this characteristic can be found by referencing the Chapter on Self-Hypnosis). Simply stated, there is more conscious effort to put someone else under hypnosis than is required to simply lie back and imagine the suggestions that another person is formulating for us. Therefore, any AASCs listed in the table that involve an operator, therapist, or instructor, such as creative visualization, biofeedback, or guided imagery, can often bring a person into a deeper level of hypnosis. Additionally, the wider the combination of techniques involved in achieving an ASC, the deeper the level. For this reason, because hypnosis usually combines many techniques from various AASCs, it often maintains the advantage of putting the willing subject into the deeper levels of trance more consistently.

Finally, the reader may consider that many of the ASCs listed in the table are on a continuum and may overlap. For example, daydreaming may be voluntarily or consciously applied to ourselves for a predetermined purpose; however, most individuals (the norm) experience this phenomena unconsciously on a regular basis, which thereby generally classifies it as a UASC. For example, many individuals with illness are taught to daydream with their eyes closed in the visual imagery practices that take place in most hospitals today through the nursing staff. Coincidentally, the most effective hypnotic inductions include combinations of visual imagery, biofeedback, guided imagery, progressive relaxation, meditation, NLP, and often indirect forms of prayer.

A certified hypnotherapist who had completed my training program had advertised her services as a certified hypnotherapist to some fundamental religious sects and, as a result, was scrutinized and interviewed by a popular Christian university newspaper. She caused quite a controversy over its ethical use in this population, so she subsequently put the reporter into a state of hypnosis, in order to prove its safety and efficacy. Afterward, the article quoted him saying that hypnosis "felt like being prayed over." So does this mean that prayer is hypnosis? The answer is *yes* and *no*. *Yes*—we must consider using synonymous labels for the phenomena of ASCs because of the interchangeable techniques involved in achieving them. The labels may be different, but the effect of achieving an altered state of consciousness is the same. And *no*, though we are achieving the same state, the subjective experience that occurs in the mind's eye is often very different from one ASC to the next. To further understand this concept, let's compare Applied ASCs below in Table 1-2.

Comparing Applied Altered States of Consciousness

The techniques applied to produce an ASC lie on a spectrum ranging from physical to psychic. Some AASCs have high degrees of physically oriented relaxation techniques used to induce the ASC, while other AASCs have more mental, or psychic, relaxation tools. I have listed below all of the AASCs for the purpose of achieving a methods comparison in Table 1-2.

Table 1-2
Classifications of Applied Altered States of Consciousness

	Physical	Psychic
Meditation	Avg.	Avg.
Biofeedback	High	Low
Transcendental Meditation	Avg.	High
Prayer	Low	High
Creative Visualization	Low	High
NLP	Low	High
Reiki	High	Low
Guided Imagery	Low	High
Guided Meditation	Avg.	Avg.
Yoga	High	Low
Progressive Relaxation	High	Low
Self-Hypnosis	High	High
Hypnotherapy	High	High

In the AASCs above, we recognize that there is a combination of physical and psychic, or mental, techniques used to achieve the altered state. Notice the extremes, such as Creative Visualization having a high amount of psychic and a low amount of physical activity. Likewise, we see that Progressive Relaxation involves a high amount of physical and a low amount of psychic activity. As we look at Self-Hypnosis and Hypnotherapy, we notice the unique characteristic of high amounts of both psychic and physical induction tools used to achieve the altered state. (This will be expounded upon in the chapter on induction).

These classifications would accurately presuppose that Nurses, Physicians, Ministers, Stress Therapists, Massage Therapists, Athletes, Motivational Speakers, NLP Practitioners, Reiki Therapists, Yoga and Meditation Instructors all use a form of hypnosis in order to achieve their purposes. Again, there are different labels for the same state. Medical research performed by Korn and Johnson resulted in a list of AASCs, similar to that in Table 1-1, and showed that "there is great overlap between what is labeled hypnosis and what is labeled otherwise."[3] In addition, hypnosis was consistently the most reliable method for achieving an altered state commonly referred to by Herbert Benson, MD, as "the relaxation response." Korn and Johnson also found that using an ASC twice a day provided the best mental and physical stress relief, and therefore, an optimal state of health and wellness.

Milton Erickson said that forms of waking hypnosis (or what we refer to as UASC) include meditation, story telling, and reading a book. It appears that anything with a story line is a form of hypnosis, because the subconscious mind works in a sequential fashion to draw on the mind's eye experience, or imagination. All ASCs are forms of hypnosis, from watching television to engaging in prayer, and hypnosis combines methods from many other ASCs, which makes it the best way to enter into an ASC. Additionally, hypnotic techniques have become more standardized than the other ASCs, and are therefore more easily and effectively utilized by professionals and their clients.

The Textbook Definition of Hypnosis

Hypnosis is an altered state of consciousness which lies between the waking state and sleep. It is generally brought about in an individual by the use of a combination of concentration, relaxation, suggestion, and expectation.

Transpersonal Definition of Hypnosis

As students of hypnotherapy, we are involved in *hypnotism,* which is defined as the *study of hypnosis.* James Braid, known as the *father of hypnosis,* coined the term "hypnosis" after the Greek word *hypnos,* which means "sleep." In Greek Mythology, the god of sleep was known as *Hypnos.* The word "therapy" is derived from the Latin word *therapeau,* which means "God's work." Therefore, if we were to take historical derivatives into consideration, we could technically define the word *hypnotherapy* as *God's work through a sleep-like state.*

Hypnosis and hypnotherapy are embedded within our culture, not only through various holistic arts that a variety of modern day holistic health practitioners make available to the public, but also through simple daily living when ASCs occur spontaneously and unconsciously. Therefore, a broad definition must be considered when the student of hypnotherapy ponders its definition. New uses for hypnotic states are being developed over time, and new devices (computers, etc.) and behaviors are triggering more hypnogogic states within our every-day life in our increasingly automated society; so the definition of hypnosis is likely to become more broad in the coming age. The profession of hypnotherapy is burgeoning, and there will be even more uses for various hypnotherapeutic approaches in the future.

Chapter 2

History and Evolution

It is important to keep in mind that the history of hypnosis is affected by the historical evolution of science and medicine. Therefore, in order to gain a greater understanding of this history, the student of hypnosis may want to do further research into the history of science and medicine, which is beyond the scope of this text. Nonetheless, describing the evolution of hypnosis may provide the reader generalizations for specific phenomena that have been believed to contain elements of hypnosis and suggestion during certain eras in human evolution.

As we look back, we can cite many uses for altered states, or hypnosis, which border on mysticism. Hypnosis dates back thousands of years to ancient religious practices, such as the sleep temples in Egypt and ancient tribal rituals like fire walking and body piercing. It has played roles in the eras of mesmerism and magnetism, the pioneering of psychoanalysis, and in the latter part of the twentieth century when psychosomatics and the "placebo effect" were used for pinpointing scientific results in medical studies. Now, psychosomatics are gaining more credibility as an important variable in people's ability to improve their illnesses. As we move into the twenty-first century, society is becoming more aware of research showing the importance of the relationship between the mind and body, or how our thoughts affect us. As a result, individuals are taking more responsibility for their health, which is paving the way for suggestive and energetic therapies to be studied and practiced independent of other mainstream professions. What I will attempt to clarify in this chapter is a historical frame of thought passed down through the ages, relative to hypnosis, up to the present era.

With the history of hypnosis, I will indirectly be discussing the various eras in the evolution of thought and reason. Mystical phenomena *resulting* from a state of hypnosis will be expounded upon in the chapter on mysticism. There are numerous writings by various researchers in the field of hypnosis containing many varying opinions on the subject of hypnotic phenomena. The single common denominator among most of the writings on the subject is that suggestion is void of spiritual intervention. Instead, I attempt to show a distinction between divine intervention through religious practices and the use of suggestion, and when both or either may be at work. We often question which produces the result. Is it a higher power that created us which affects our mind, body, and spiritual purpose, or is the belief in a higher power simply a concept that our mind and body respond to when a healing or transformation takes place? Perhaps it is that we are created in the image of God, and so God exists within each of us, within the power of our minds, and this is why beliefs are so important in healing. Maybe it is all of the above. Either way, it is important for the transpersonal hypnotherapist to keep these possibilities in mind when examining the history of hypnosis relative to healing.

History of Hypnosis

Before we explore the history of hypnosis, I would like to emphasize that this section does not include certain subcategories of hypnosis that other hypnosis researchers traditionally include, such as exorcism or energy healing. In other writings, these are classified under the umbrella of hypnotic suggestion. I do not share that opinion; however, I do consistently teach from the perspective that hypnotherapy is much more effective if we are operating from within the client's belief system. In addition, the concepts of beliefs and imagination are segmented and expounded upon in subsequent chapters, in order to take a more thorough look into the clinical and transpersonal aspects of each concept.

It is my opinion that externally originated healing (healing from a higher power) *does* exist, in addition to energy healing practices (such as Reiki, Magnetism, and the like); and suggestion, which may be classified under internally originated healing, also exists (more on the origin of healing in the next chapter). With this in mind, it will be important that we ponder the forces at work under the myriad of techniques used throughout the history of hypnosis. While contemplating these, I suggest considering multiple possibilities for the labels given to describe various hypnotic or suggestive phenomena.

Paracelsus (1493-1541) was among the *first to heal the sick with magnets*. His emphasis was on the magnetic flow of energy within what he called the astral body—a metaphysical body and integral part of a person's spirit. Once this astral body was put in balance with magnets, an individual's disease or illness would disappear. This view was shared by many during this era, such as Glocenius, Burgrove, Helnotius, Fludd, Kircher, Van Helmont, Balthazar Gracian, Porta, and Maxwell.

William Maxwell (writing in 1679) was a Scottish physician who also adhered to the magnetic healing theory but also embraced the concept that a vital, universal spirit affected all human beings. Later in his work, he hypothesized that *imagination and suggestion* influenced a person's ability to heal.

Maximilian Hell (1720-1792) was a Viennese Jesuit priest and astronomer who was the first to become famous for producing healings through the direct application of *metal plates* to the naked body. He conducted his work under similar beliefs as William Maxwell, hypothesizing that there were spiritual variables that occurred in magnetic healing.

Franz Anton Mesmer (1734-1815) was an Austrian physician from Vienna who, according to some writings, first took an interest in metal plate healings through hearing of Father Hell's work. He hypothesized that optimum health depended on the balance of a "universal fluid" within the body, which emanated from the stars and the planets. He called this effect *animal magnetism*. In 1773, he presented his thesis, "The influence of the Stars and Planets as Curative Powers," to the Faculty of Medicine at the University of Vienna. In order to cure the sick, Mesmer felt that the magnetic flow of the fluid within the patient should be adjusted with *magnetism*. He began by making passes with magnets over the affected areas of the sick with astounding results. Consequently, this new healing method eventually brought him mass notoriety as a great healer.

Most researchers agree that Mesmer was greatly influenced by Father Hell's work, but F.A. Patties' research also revealed that Mesmer studied the writings of the English Physician Richard Mead (1673-1754), who was inspired by the research of his patient, Sir Isaac Newton. Mesmer was inspired by Newton's study and explanation of natural laws affecting living systems.[4] Another popular story claims that Mesmer stumbled across a street magician's show where lodestones or magnets were used to demonstrate that he could make a spectator do his bidding by touching him with a magnet. It is reported that suggestion was the key to performing this act, but Mesmer believed magnets actually had a power of their own. Regardless of how Mesmer was influenced to do his work, it is certain that his contributions are highly valued.

Eventually, Mesmer developed a sizeable following. In order to handle the enormous crowds, he devised a mass healing approach called the *baquet*- a large tub filled with iron filings from which magnetized iron rods protruded, and thirty or more persons could participate at the same time, clutching the rods. Sometimes they were joined together with cords. As Mesmer magnetized each person by touching him or her with a glass rod, he or she would often go into convulsions or hysteria. Sometimes it would take one treatment, and at other times it took several, in order to experience a cure. Later, he hypothesized that animal magnetism was in everything, humans, animals, and inanimate objects, and that all he needed to do was pass his hands over somebody to produce the same results.

Again, in order to handle the crowds, he offered a new

method for healing. He contended that he transferred his animal magnetism into a nearby tree, and it was there that many thousands of people were healed by touching it. Some historical records suggest that by the latter part of the eighteenth century, Mesmer had up to three thousand patients seeking treatment each day!

Because of his popularity, he and his methods drew attention from the medical profession. As a result, Mesmer invited the French Academy of Science to Vienna to study his methods. In 1784, a commission was set up with nine members that included the American diplomat Benjamin Franklin, the French chemist Antoine-Laurent Lavoisier, Doctor Guillotin—the physician who invented the guillotine, and a popular botanist of the time named Antoine-Laurent de Jussieu. When they went to the place where Mesmer worked his magic, they watched him heal a boy with his methods. Mesmer told Johnny that he would be healed if he sat under a nearby tree. He did as he was told and was thereby cured. After studying events such as these, the commission agreed that miraculous healings were taking place; however, they concluded that it was from the use of imagination and suggestion.

Thereafter, magnetism was debunked, and the new title for the phenomenon became *Mesmerism*. Thus, an end quickly came to the belief in magnetism, and Mesmer became labeled a quack. Deeply discouraged, he left France in 1785, traveled throughout Europe, and retired in a small town in Germany. Near the end of his life, he relocated to Switzerland where he died in poverty and seclusion in 1815.

Marquis de Puysegur (1781-1825) was a French military officer and follower of Mesmer. One day, while he was applying magnetism to a 24 year old shepherd, the subject fell into a deep peaceful sleep. The young man was able to talk in a slurred fashion and open his eyes, but forgot everything he had said after he was awakened. Puysegur called this "artificial somnambulism," now referred to as *hypnotic amnesia,* and held the view that mesmerism was a psychological phenomenon.

Petetin was also a follower of Mesmer and discovered the effect of *hypnotic catalepsy*. After he magnetized subjects, they were unable to move any part of their body until told to do so.

Barbarin, another follower of Mesmer, magnetized without paraphernalia and his followers called themselves Barbarinists. However, in Sweden and Germany they were called *spiritualists*, because the cures were thought to be acts of God.

Joseph Philippe Francois Deleuze (1753-1835) was the librarian of the Royal Botanical and Zoological Gardens when he went to personally witness Mesmer's work, at which time he wrote:

"In one room, under the influence of rods issuing from tubs filled with large bottles — the said rods applied upon different parts of the subjects' bodies — the most extraordinary scenes took place daily. Sardonic laughter, piteous moans and torrents of tears burst forth on all sides. The subjects were thrown back in spasmodic jerks, the respirations sounded like death rattles, and terrifying symptoms were exhibited. Suddenly, the actors of these strange performances would frantically or rapturously rush towards each other, either rejoicing and embracing, or thrusting away their neighbors with every appearance of horror.

Another room was padded, and presented a different spectacle. There, women beat their heads against the padded walls or rolled on the cushion-covered floor in fits of suffocation. In the midst of the panting, quivering throng, Mesmer, dressed in a lilac coat, moved about, halting in front of the most violently excited, and gazing steadily into their eyes, while he held both their hands in his, bringing the middle fingers into immediate contact to establish the communication. At another moment he would, by a motion of open hands and extended fingers, operate with the great current, crossing and uncrossing his arm with wonderful rapidity to make the final passes."

Sometime thereafter, as he studied and practiced Mesmerism on his own, Deleuze discovered that suggestions given to the patient while under the Mesmeric state would be carried out later in the waking state. This would later be known as his primary contribution to the field of hypnosis. Today, this is referred to as *post hypnotic suggestion*. While he was a fluidist, he thought Mesmerism to be a psychological phenomenon.

Jose Custodio de Faria (1755-1819) was a Portuguese priest who came to Paris from India and gave public demonstrations in 1814 and 1815 on what he referred to as "lucid sleep." His theory was that the cures were not due to magnetism but to "the expectancy and cooperation of the subject." He discovered that the *subject must be willing* to carry out the suggestions while under the Mesmeric state, which is still valid today relative to hypnosis.

Récamier, in 1821, was the first to conduct operations on patients who were somnambulistic and under the Mesmeric state. This is the *first recorded use of hypnoanesthesia.*
Another French physician by the name of **Hippolyte Cloquet** demonstrated a breast operation using Mesmerism in front of the French Academy of Medicine in 1829. At that time, an American physician by the name of **Wheeler** performed a nasal polypectomy using Mesmerism. This was the first reported use of *hypnoanesthesia in the United States.*

John Elliotson (1791-1868) was a surgeon who invented the stethoscope and *popularized hypnoanesthesia* in England. At the time, he was the professor of medicine at the University of London hospital. After a short time of using "Mesmerism" for surgery, he was labeled a quack and an impostor. Both the university and the church opposed its use, so he resigned. As a fearless scientist, he published "The Zoist," a journal that reported numerous painless operations and other Mesmeric phenomena.

James Esdaile (1808-1859) was a Scottish surgeon who practiced Mesmerism in India from 1840 to 1850. He reported hundreds of painless operations. This eventually became known as the *Esdaile Method for Hypnoanesthesia.* Other local physicians also began using the method, and the mortality rate dropped from 50% to 5%, in contrast to chemo-anesthesia. By 1849, physicians in the United States were starting to recommend Mesmerism for pain relief during surgery.

James Braid (1795-1860) is known as the "father of hypnosis." He was a Scottish physician who, after attending a demonstration by LaFontaine, the Swiss magnetizer, scoffed at the idea of the energy-healing position of magnetism. Instead, he contended that expectation influenced a person's susceptibility to suggestion. Unfortunately, he coined the terms "hypnotism" and "hypnosis" after the Greek word *hypnos*, which means *sleep*. Later he realized that hypnosis was not sleep, but by then the term had already stuck to the phenomenon. As a scientist, he began experimenting with *eye fixation*. He believed that a tiring of the eyes, by paralyzing the optic nerve centers, would produce hypnosis.

Jean-Martin Charcot (1825-1893), a neurologist who worked at Salpetrier, an insane asylum, believed hypnosis was pathological, causing hysteria. With the aid of **Doctor Burcq**, a French physician, he briefly revived "Magnetism." Burcq was an experimentalist who studied the work of Mesmer and began using metal plates on the mentally ill. As a result of strapping metal plates to the body, a process he called metaloscopy, sensation of anesthetized patients was restored. While theorizing hypnosis was pathological in nature, Charcot instituted the *Salpetrier School of Hypnosis.* Known as the Salpetrier School of Thought, this theory was later refuted by the studies done by Ambroise-Auguste Liebeault and Hippolyte Bernheim.

Ambroise-Auguste Liebeault (1823-1904) was a French physician who practiced in a small town outside of Nancy. He used hypnosis for a variety of medical conditions and, with behavior modification, had remarkable success curing organic diseases. He wrote a book on his results called *Du Sommeil,* but only one copy was sold. Fees were charged for those who desired treatment with drugs, but to avoid being labeled a charlatan, hypnotherapy treatments were free. He later became known as the father of *suggestive-therapeutic hypnosis.*

Together with **Hippolyte Bernheim** (1837-1919), a neurologist from Nancy, France, they developed the Nancy School of Thought, which emphasized hypnosis as being a psychological phenomenon. Before this, Bernheim was a professor at the Medical School of Nancy and a strict proponent of drug therapy. After a patient who had sciatica left him for Liebeault's hypnotherapy treatments and was cured with hypnotic suggestion, Bernheim set out to prove him a quack. However, after studying and becoming fascinated with his methods, Bernheim became a proponent of hypnotherapy and a devotee of Liebeault. Soon thereafter, the *Nancy School of Hypnosis* was born and became very famous, treating over 12,000 patients over the life of its operation. The school emphasized suggestion and suggestibility as naturally occurring psychological aspects of hypnosis and the mind.

Sigmund Freud (1856-1939), known as the "pioneer of psychoanalysis," studied with Liebeault and Bernheim at the Nancy School of Hypnosis. After his training, he avoided the use of hypnosis, because he felt that he could not produce the effect consistently in many of his patients. In addition, he could not get those he *did* hypnotize to a sufficient depth. Most investigators would agree that Freud's very basic techniques, and therefore his abilities using hypnosis, were very limited. Eventually, his use of hypnosis was limited to those whom he could hypnotize successfully. He also contended that the hypnotized client's resistances were stripped too quickly, in comparison to the slower methods used in psychotherapy. In addition, he surmised that cures from hypnosis were only temporary.

Most investigators agree that he had difficulty incorporating hypnosis into the specific therapeutic approach that he favored, and that his hypnotherapy skills, eye fixation for example, were very mundane. He later abandoned hypnosis for *psychoanalysis, free association, and dream induction* with the belief that *catharsis,* a state he referred to as a form of therapeutic purification, was more effective when it was consciously triggered over a number of years, rather than being unconsciously triggered through short-term hypnotherapy sessions.

Although most researchers today disagree with Freud's findings regarding hypnosis, credit must be given to him for making some wonderful contributions to understanding archetypal or universal aspects of the mind. His theory called *psychic determinism* hypothesized that a symptom displayed on the surface had a deeper cause that could be found within the unconscious levels of the mind. Once this cause was uncovered, the symptoms disappeared.

Another great contribution was *repetition compulsion*, where a problem will cyclically be recreated and will rematerialize in a person's life until the patient's responses to it change. Once the problem is responded to differently, it is eliminated from recurring. A spiritual view of the repetition compulsion theory suggests that life lessons occur because of the restructuring of the environment by the collective unconscious (as Carl Jung referred to it), which is a sum total of individual human thoughts converging on the physical material plane.

The concept of *patterns* was also mentioned by Edgar Cayce in other contexts, such as the need to repeat certain behavior patterns so that individual entities, or human beings, could learn life lessons. (See more under Edgar Cayce and Carl Jung.) Without patterns, everything would be perceived as occurring for the first time. In other words, we would be on a single trial learning curve, and everything would therefore be almost incomprehensible. Although patterns are necessary for learning, it is the dysfunctional habit patterns that drive people to seek therapy.

Although many of Freud's theories are viewed as being outdated, or ridiculous, as in the cases of his sexual theories, he made some great discoveries. Most of his greatest discoveries and theories that are still popular were the result of his years of experimentation with hypnosis.

Pierre Janet (1859-1947) worked under Freud. His contribution to hypnosis is known as the *Theory of Dissociation*. This is where a person under hypnosis ignores what is happening in the present circumstances and simultaneously recall the past. In other words, the client mentally leaves the present awareness and enters another reality, such as in hypnotic regression. Personality exploration under hypnosis was used extensively by Janet for therapeutic purposes.

The **American Medical Association** (1958) endorsed the use of hypnosis as a *valid therapeutic tool*. At that time, there was a movement which encouraged all medical schools across the United States to offer hypnosis training to their medical students.

Therefore, in the early 1960s, hypnosis education was part of virtually every medical school's curriculum. Hypnosis for childbirth became a viable option for expectant mothers in the 1960s and 1970s proving notable success in producing comfortable levels of hypnoanesthesia. We may notice, when conversing with physicians who graduated from medical school during that time, that most of these individuals had training in hypnosis as part of their education.

Edgar Cayce (1877-1945) was often referred to as the *sleeping prophet*, because he would undergo a sleep-like state, hypnosis, to read the mind, body, and spiritual forces at work in the lives of his subjects. The subject could be thousands of miles away. Yet, after applying a state of self-hypnosis, he could accurately diagnose and recommend a cure for the illness in a person's body. This astounded many physicians of that time, who did not have available x-ray and other modern diagnostic tools. After some time, his readings focused on the mental makeup of his clients, and then the spiritual purpose for which they incarnated. His readings included deep aspects of the human plight, reincarnation, nonphysical planes of existence, and future prophecy. He is respected by many for his prophecies which, according to some researchers who have investigated their historical validity, are approximately 85% accurate.

Like Freud, Edgar Cayce referred to patterns, or "cycles," that exist mentally and then rematerialize in the physical environment for the purpose of learning. Cayce also referred to the concept of *karma* in many of his readings. In most eastern religions, karma means "carry over" from one life to the next, as in reincarnation. Although health readings were mostly what surfaced in the beginning, it was in later years that his readings taught concepts of reincarnation, and his *life readings* became very popular.

His life readings involved a process by which Cayce accessed a place he called the *akashic records* of human beings in order to read their past lives, their current mental emotional and physical condition, and their future options. The akashic records held most of the important information regarding an individual. This place is thought by many, myself included, to be the same place as Carl Jung's "collective unconscious" (see Jung below). Here exist the nonphysical records of every living thing's past, present, and probable future—(according to Cayce, intuiting the future involved probabilities that were based on current individual and collective thought, and could therefore be changed).

Hypnosis was important to Edgar Cayce, particularly earlier in his career when he lost his voice and used his unique state of self-hypnosis, combined with readings, to cure himself of the condition. Subsequently, he consistently entered a state of self-hypnosis to perform readings for thousands of individuals who requested them, and as a result, many illnesses and diseases were helped or cured.

Interestingly, Edgar Cayce recommended hypnotherapy sessions to his subjects only on a handful of occasions. Most of the recommendations for his clients' problems involved natural remedies and mental enlightenments. Perhaps this is because of the era in which the readings were given (the early 1900s). Certainly, the level of hypnotherapeutic education has dramatically evolved since then, resulting in more advanced levels of hypnotherapeutic treatments. Nonetheless, Cayce's contributions to the field of hypnosis are destined to become more relevant and more appreciated with time.

Carl Jung (1875-1961), was at first looked at as an oddity within the mental health circles of his era. However, by the 1970s, his theories become most popular and were taught at virtually every college campus within the United States. One of his primary contributions was *archetypes*. These were considered common forms of thought. Individuals automatically contributed their thoughts to, and extracted various thoughts from, a place he referred to as the *"collective unconscious."*

This was similar to Cayce's theory of the akashic records in that there was a storehouse of memories from every living being. This storehouse is supposedly nonphysical and responsible for our images that surface in dreams and imagination. According to Jung, these images may contain deep psychological traits of the dreamer/imaginer. In addition, these thoughts, which are from the collective area, are theorized to have also originated from other people and may be involved in "intuition." Carl Jung documented several cases of intuition between him and his clients, even imply-ing that intuition was an important variable within the therapeutic process.

If we were to further explore the concept of collective thought, we could hypothesize that some of the "past lives" that individuals encounter while in a state of hypnosis could be attrib-uted to plucking a memory from the collective unconscious. Then again, it could be just what the client sometimes believes it to be, a memory that was actually experienced by the client in another lifetime at some point in the earth plane.

With some reflection, it is easy to see that Carl Jung's con-tributions to hypnosis are metaphysical in nature. The origin of thought and its collective influence is more relevant now than ever before. Considering the current awareness of psychic manifestation, a new look at Jungian material could lead to greater metaphysical insights.

Milton H. Erickson (1901-1980) was a psychiatrist, psy-chologist, and a great hypnotherapist who helped the practice of hypnotherapy become more accepted by the medical and mental health communities, and the general public. He combined the two primary schools of thought (pathological verses psychological) and popularized the concept that hypnosis was "a naturally oc-curring psychophysiological phenomenon." He believed that each of us enters into hypnosis several times per day, a phenomenon he referred to as *waking hypnosis*. Some examples of this include common activities such as watching television, reading a book, meditating, daydreaming, story telling, driving an automobile, and more.

Many of his profound cures were due to telling his clients stories in which they could imagine being one of the characters. Ideas were often shared within the story that were symbolic of the client's condition. This is referred to as *metaphor construction*. In one case[5], the client, who was an alcoholic, told Erickson that he didn't think he could stop drinking. Erickson states, "I send alcoholic patients to AA..., but this one was a wonderful chal-lenge to accept." As a result of careful listening, Dr. Erickson gave his patient a "doctor's order" to go to the Botanical Gardens and sit among the "cacti that can survive three years without water, without rain. And do a lot of thinking."

Many years later a woman came to see him and said, "Dr. Erickson, you knew me when I was three years old. I moved to California when I was three years old. Now I am in Phoenix and I came to see what kind of a man you were—what you looked like." Dr. Erickson, with his usual rapport-building language, responded, "Take a good look, and I'm curious to know why you want to look at me." She said, "Any man who would send an alcoholic out to the Botanical Gardens to look around, to learn how to get around without alcohol, and have it work, is the kind of man I want to see! My mother and father have been sober ever since you sent my father out there." Apparently, when she was three years old, the time Erickson worked with her father, he quit drinking and got a prosperous job with a magazine company in California.

This story is a beautiful example of *indirect suggestion*, where a client is entranced by his problem, naturally going into the altered state. Erickson often utilized this waking trance-state and suggested a specific idea at the moment of suggestibility, which dramatically altered the realities of the problem; and as a result, the client stopped drinking. Often, these indirect suggestions were of an enlightening nature to the current perceptual realities of the client, and they would be planted in the client's mind as the next step toward change.

Erickson was also known as the *master of rapport*. He believed that the therapist could not help a client change, until he or she was experiencing the client's model of the world, thus developing rapport. In essence, by identifying with the client's problem, he would produce a mind sharing effect known as rapport. The client would feel as though he or she were understood. This is what I refer to as sharing space with the client. Rapport is necessary, in order to facilitate new perceptual realities within the client. It is the most important factor in creating a successful induction, according to Erickson. Thus, transformation and behavior change are the result most often achieved by gaining rapport.

Reframing was also emphasized throughout Erickson's work. This is a way to help a client re-perceive his or her problem within a whole new light. Often, replacing one word for another when feeding back a sentence stated by the client makes a big difference in shifting the client's perceptions. If a client claims that he or she has a "fear," for example, a therapist may be able to suggest that he or she is simply wise to be "cautious" by saying, "Being cautious is okay, so let's let go of the fear, shall we?" I tried reframing with a gymnast that was afraid of landing on her head when doing a double back flip; changing the word "fear" to "caution," in combination with suggestive therapy, worked beautifully.

Much of Neurolinguistic Programming (NLP) was derived from **Richard Bandler's** and **John Grinder's** observations of Erickson's techniques. These gentlemen may be credited for being the creators of NLP. Grinder specialized in the study of language and Bandler specialized in the study of subconscious processes. The client interview methods taught in this book include NLP, or Ericksonian methodology, as a foundation for eliciting and changing an individual's motivations. The Ericksonian techniques in this text are very helpful in producing trance and change, but a separate course in Ericksonian hypnosis or Neurolinguistic Programming may also be useful.

In reference to clinical practicality, it is important to consider the era in which Dr. Erickson practiced, in order to put these authoritarian methods in proper perspective. In other words, how many people do we know in today's age who would go stand in an atrium of cacti as a result of a "doctor's order?" This is an example of an extreme authoritarian style of hypnotherapy. The permissive approach is widely preferred by hypnotherapists and clients today, so many of the authoritarian methods for which Erickson gained notoriety have become outdated. Nonetheless, the tools that created extraordinary transformations are still relevant and often highly effective when taught and utilized in the appropriate contexts.

Transpersonal Hypnotherapy (Present)—The word *transpersonal* means the *crossing of body, mind, and spirit.* It assumes that humans operate on all three levels, or that the mind, body, and spirit of an individual affect each other. Because human beings are of spiritual origin, this important component of the therapeutic paradigm should not be overlooked within the practice of hypnotherapy. With this variable in operation, client sessions proceed more rapidly, and the various clinical tools of hypnotherapy are more transformative. Transpersonal hypnotherapy is a frame of thought in the field of hypnotherapy that embraces the clinical aspects of hypnosis, but also adds the client's higher dimensional realities to therapeutic interventions when deemed appropriately beneficial to the client.

When a transpersonal hypnotherapist is posed the philosophical question, "Are we physical beings trying to have a spiritual experience, or are we spiritual beings trying to have a physical experience?", he or she is sure to respond with the latter. Transpersonal hypnotherapy involves the awareness of the spirit (or soul) of the individual experiencing the therapy in either a subtle or obvious way, depending on the client's needs. It assumes that individuals are on some type of path to discover and engage in a higher good. Good is the locus for the inner scale of comparison in conscience. This inherent inner component (human beings being inherently good at the core) allows for an awareness of life's contrasts for the purpose of learning and progress. It also theorizes that hypnosis is the "bridge" between the three primary components of human consciousness, and that these components (body, mind, and spirit) may be accessed through the use of altered states of consciousness, hypnosis being the most effective. Hypnosis is believed to have the ability, simply by itself, to create greater self awareness, self-understanding, and a holistic body-mind-spirit connectedness.

As we ponder the history of hypnosis, it may become apparent that eras of human thought coincide with the evolutionary understanding of hypnosis and its application. In our current era, we can see that altered-state therapies—hypnosis, magnetism, energy-healing, and transpersonalism—are gaining in credibility. Rather than just being written off by science as having a temporary "placebo effect," the practices of alternative and complementary therapies are given their proper place in healing. The era of authoritarianism is over, and the more permissive approach, which includes an openness toward transpersonalism, is "in" by popular public demand.

The trend of individuals taking responsibility for their health care needs is here to stay. The validity for the coexistence of medical science and alternative and preventive health care practices continues to gain more momentum each year. There will be many more flowers blooming from the stalks of this trend in the future, and transpersonal hypnotherapists are providing some of the main branches for growth, understanding, and transformation.

Chapter 3

Mysticism, Intention, and Suggestion

Several hundred years before the time of Christ, tribal medicine men, witch doctors, and religious leaders had practiced forms of hypnosis and altered states of consciousness in order to affect the mind, body, or spiritual realms of thought or being. These practices included chants, rhythmical beats (drums), rituals, and ceremonial practices which often produced sleep-like states that resulted in miraculous cures. As early as 3000 B.C., *sleep temples* in ancient Greece and Egypt were used for healing. Curative suggestions were repeatedly given to an individual while he or she was sleeping in the temple through the night. In the morning, "voila!"— in most cases, the "Gods" did their job, or was it the use of suggestions and affirmations that produced the results?

Through the ages, astounding hypnotic practices, such as fire-walking, were used in many ancient cultures. Even in the United States today, fire-walking is popular for those who wish to experience the power of the mind and its ability to overcome physical and mental limitations. In order to accomplish this feat, individuals often repeat an affirmation, sing, or chant, thereby entering into a hypnotic or altered state. With the proper mind-set, they walk on the fire without getting burned.

In the time of Christ, many "miracles" through divine intervention of a spiritual, mental, and physical nature transpired. It is important to note that some researchers in the field of hypnosis indicate that this phenomena was specifically a result of the power of suggestion. However, I believe that the events that have been written about in the western world's biblical text involving miraculous physiological cures, spirit depossessions, mystical intuition, or psychic ability, as well as the mental-emotional shifts resulting in those who came into contact with Christ, were a result of an energy exchange as part of his relationship to a higher power or creative source. In other words, these phenomena were not a result of suggestion in the traditional sense, but of spiritual origin. One possibility that we should embrace is that it is likely that those who were healed had indeed experienced some form of altered states of consciousness, similar to hypnosis. Yet, this does not undermine the probability that supernatural forces had been at work during the healing experience. It does appear to suggest that the altered state of consciousness coincides with the occurrence of spiritual phenomena.

In recent times, primarily the birth of the 21st century, we can see a relationship between visionaries (those who claim to see Marian and Christ apparitions) and the hypnotic state. For example, one of the most dramatic demonstrations of this was in the case where 5 children in Medjugorje, Yugoslavia, claimed to have seen and spoken with Mary, the mother of Christ. As soon as she supposedly entered the room, they dropped to their knees and began to take turns talking to what appeared to be thin air. When tested by lip readers from many different parts of the world, it was determined that the children were speaking a language of unknown origin. When they were pricked with needles, they were undisturbed; and when they had metal plates put before their eyes, their transfixed gaze was unaltered. They remained in an ecstatic state and continued to carry on conversation.

It was determined by neurological researchers using an electroencephalogram (EEG) that the children's brain waves indicated altered states of consciousness (alpha, theta, and delta). In my opinion, they were very similar to EEG readings derived from those measured on individuals in a state of hypnosis. Another similarity exists between those in a deep level of hypnosis, who generally experience anesthesia, and the anesthesia which occurs with visionaries during apparitions.

When individuals are under deep hypnosis and then pierced with a needle, they also feel nothing. As a result, we could conclude that mystical experiences generally involve an altered state of consciousness of a depth similar to that of hypnosis.

Were the children in Medjugorje experiencing figments of their imagination? In many of these cases, the possibility should be considered that the supernatural, or an outside force, is at work. There are numerous accounts of "Spiritual" healing passed down throughout history from culture to culture by way of various religious practices and ceremonies. The most powerful, well documented form of spiritual healing was seen in the times of Christ. However, over the eons, there have been many other non-Christian religious practices that have produced healing, and these should not be overlooked by hypnotherapists who work with clients from all walks of faith.

My question to students of hypnosis is the same one I have posed to myself for many years, "How does the spiritual dimension of being, (or the supernatural) given that it does exist, relate to altered states of consciousness when it comes to divine healing?" When these so called "miracles" do take place, is it the power of suggestion, our own faith, or an outside spiritual force that heals us? Those familiar with the Western biblical text can recall Christ discussing the origin of healing on several occasions. In one reported case, a woman who was hemorrhaging fought her way through the crowds to be healed. When she finally reached him, she reached out and touched his cloak and was healed instantly. J.C. then looked around to ask who touched his cloak, because he felt the energy go out from him to her. She was afraid at first and did not admit to what she had done. Then, she admitted to the act, and he said to her, "...your faith has cured you."[6]

Let's take a broader look at healing. The best resource I have ever found for describing healing from this perspective is, *The Healing Power of Faith*, by Wil Oursler. In this writing, he studied several world religions ranging from Catholicism to Native American. All of the many healing ceremonies that he studied had one thing in common. The individual who was healed did not need to have faith that it would happen beforehand. It was only necessary for the practitioner (healer, priest, shaman, minister, etc.) to have faith, in order for healing to occur. In some cases, all it took was a bystander to have the faith that a healing would occur.

According to Oursler's book, some of the best documented cases of spiritual healing that have occurred were at the Marian apparition site of Lourdes, France. In brief, the story goes like this... A girl named Bernadette was playing with her friends one day by a pig's pen which was roped off into a cave. There, she started to speak to "a lady" who called herself "the immaculate conception (of Christ)." After great persecution by the townspeople, and the local government, Bernadette's story never changed; and she persevered to meet with the apparition regularly. One day, the lady told Bernadette that a spring would come out of the ground and heal the sick. After Bernadette dug in the mud like a lunatic in front of hundreds of disbelieving locals, she ate a piece of mud and a spring began gushing forth. Mary said, "Make way for the procession," and since then, millions of people have visited this site annually, encountering various forms of healing.

Oursler's book continues to describe how a team of physicians was utilized to examine those with practically every form of illness or disease before they went into the healing pools. After they came out of the pools, those with claims of healing were examined again. If they did not have a relapse in their condition within one year, and after a one year follow-up examination, it was considered a miracle by divine intervention.

One dramatic case involved a man with an open fracture that wouldn't heal. After several months of crutches and a festering infection on an open wound, he dragged his leg onto a bus, was lectured by the bus driver for leaving blood stains there, and was dropped off at the Lourdes hospital, *Bureau De Medicales*. There, he was examined by a team of physicians, entered into the healing pools, and was examined again immediately afterward. The medical report documented an instantaneous melding of the bone and a closure of the open wound. A line where the fracture used to be was the only indication that there was a break in the leg.

Another well documented case involved a communist official who had an incurable disease. His wife told him that he should go to Lourdes. He did not have faith in anything greater than himself, nor any higher power, but he figured he didn't have anything to lose. When he got there, he met a 10 year old boy who was also dying. The boy went into the pool with no results, but when the communist went into the pool, the boy said he would pray for the man, and the man was healed.

In another example in Oursler's book, a Methodist minister who was brand new to a congregation was asked to perform the Monday night healing ceremony that the previous minister used to perform. He did not believe in the ceremony, or these types of healings, but the parishioners pressed him to do it, so he did. He said that when the whole group started praying together, there was a wave of energy in the room that was awesomely present. It went from him through the others in the room, and then back to him, as he described it. Indeed, he was surprised to witness the healings that took place that night, and he admitted that the group's higher spiritual intention was a key factor.

Another writing which documents the effects of intention and the influence of spiritual forces is Bernie Siegel's *Love, Medicine and Miracles*. Dr. Siegel, who is an oncologist, cites in a blind study that one out of two groups who were stricken with cancer were prayed for. After years of study, the group who was prayed for lived an average of ten years longer, in comparison with the group that did not receive any organized prayer.

In all these cases, it wasn't the faith of those that were ill that was necessary for obtaining a healing, but the faith and intentions of others. This is consistently documented throughout every religion studied in Oursler's writings.

The Faith Factor and Highest Intention

The key to understanding hypnotherapeutic outcomes is in the *faith factor*. In this context, "faith" is perceived opposite to the way we would normally think about it. The key to healing by external forces is not based on the client's faith, but on the practitioner's faith instead. I often state in my classes while teaching others to become transpersonally oriented hypnotherapists, "A client will only go as far as you think they can." This was also documented in Weisenhoffer's writings on clinical hypnosis in the 1950s, positively correlating faith and results from hypnosis. Therefore, hypnotherapists, or for that matter all practitioners who desire change for their clients, must believe that anything is possible, in order to increase their results. This is what I call the *highest intention*. One way of tapping into the highest intention is to imagine, with a higher or meditative focus, the greatest possible result for specific clients. This way of thinking gives the client room to go as far into change and transformation as he or she desires, plus some.

Think of it this way. If Jill, my smoking client, asks me if I really think she can quit smoking, and I say, "Well, I think you might be able to. You have a 70% chance of success." It is likely that Jill will imagine herself falling into the 30% range that is unsuccessful, because smokers try an average of four times before quitting permanently. This statistic includes other programs in addition to hypnosis. She may quit, but she also may not; because we must factor into the equation my 30% doubt, in addition to her doubts too. If her doubts are even stronger than mine, then the faith factor is even lower when run through the *faith factor equation* for predetermining results.

In order to understand this equation, let's assume that faith falls on a scale of 1 to 10 with 1 being the lowest amount of faith and 10 being the highest. If my faith as practitioner is 10 and Jill's is 5, then the faith factor equation's sum is an average of the two, or 7.5, which equals 75% [(10+5)/2=7.5]. Jill, without the help of spiritual forces, has about a 75% chance of becoming a nonsmoker.

Without getting into a lot of detail as to the "how to" concepts of Milton Erickson's work, it can be emphasized under this section that Erickson's high level of faith influenced the faith factor and therefore the success of his sessions. Regardless of where his clients were in their faith, and regardless of the mental problem, he believed that his clients could change quickly and effectively; and therefore they did, sometimes instantaneously. After a while,

Erickson became known as a magnificent therapist and healer, which increased the faith factor of his clients. Simultaneously, this increased Erickson's faith, which raised the percentage of the entire faith factor. The result was consistent transformation. Beliefs were shifted more positively by both parties, which exponentially elevated the faith factor on each side of the equation. This effect tends to increase results over time, because of the effect I call *faith transference*, whereby each party's faith gets stronger over time because of the faith of the other party. A "faith loop," as we might refer, obviously exists.

It is best for the practitioner to be working out of the highest intention, because it is the easiest way to affect change. The absolute highest intention is a 10 on the faith scale, where every practitioner should be over time. New hypnotherapists may need to see the miraculous results of hypnotherapy, before building their faith variable; but this generally does not take long. I believe that anything is possible, so why not imagine that everyone, all of our clients, can be successful? Transpersonal hypnotherapists should believe in this, and then watch it happen more often.

As we read about the metaphysical aspects of therapy, we need to keep in mind that the vehicle we use to create change is awesomely powerful just by itself. We are using what I refer to as the *divine enlightened state*. Many visionaries, healers, and prophets, including St. Bernadette and Edgar Cayce, have experienced altered states during their periods of enlightenment. Because spiritual experiences take place in the altered state, the state of hypnosis, the transpersonal hypnotherapist has a wonderfully powerful resource to create positive change. With the proper intention, the hypnosis session therefore brings to it forces similar to that of prayer.

The greatest power that I have ever experienced is group collective intention. What is meant by this is the combined highest intentions of individuals that are grouped together for the purpose of healing and change. People may experience this effect in prayer groups, therapy groups, personal growth training courses, hypnotherapy training courses and the like. Often, in transpersonal hypnotherapy courses, the collective energy gets so strong with the combined beliefs of each of the students , that people change as much from the collective group intentions as they do from the hypnotherapy techniques, and even more so when including the highest intention, or God source.

It has been said before, by possibly the greatest teacher and healer of all time, J.C., that all things are possible through God; and those with faith could move mountains. If we give credibility to this, and we include our individual conceptualization of what or who God is in our intention for our clients, then in actuality, anything *is* possible! If our intention is high enough when working toward healing or change, then we are not only holding space for it to occur, but we are also including an energetic level request to have spiritual forces influence the hypnotherapy sessions. In addition to these effects, of course, we want to use all of our internally based resources from our education and experience.

There are two key effects that increase the success of our methods: our intention as hypnotherapist; and our calling on higher forces. Each of us uses unique channels in order to tap the latter.

Two Ways to Add Spiritual Forces to Sessions

There are two primary ways that spiritual forces may be added to the equation of change:

1) The first way involves the therapist asking his or her higher power(s) to assist them, before entering into the "sacred space," (therapy office). Personally, I like to pray a portion of the St. Francis of Assisi prayer, as follows:

"Make me an instrument of your peace, so that only the highest good will prevail this day and every day for me and my clients. Allow me to do your will."

2) The second method involves hypnotherapists clearing themselves before working with clients at the beginning of the day. This can be done by giving all personal or professional problems up to a higher source, during a self-hypnosis session, of which we would do on ourselves immediately before the session begins. This procedure is outlined in the chapter on self-hypnosis. Another benefit to clearing the self of issues beforehand is that the practitioner is not just present physically at one-hundred percent, but also mentally. The mind is not wandering, because there re-

ally aren't any distractions within. The practitioner is then able to focus all of his or her energy on the client's problematic goals, and therefore the client also focuses more on themselves.

Transpersonal hypnotherapists are both clinicians and healers. They work professionally in a clinical capacity, but also involve their spiritual resources, and those of their clients, within their sessions where it is deemed adequate and useful.

Origin of Healing Theories

In order to better understand the process of healing, we may examine two theoretical origins, internal origination and external origination . In other words, healing originates either internally or externally, but when applied in holistic therapies, they are often combined. The combination of the two is primarily dependent on the client's beliefs.

A) <u>Internal Origination</u>- All healing originates from within the self and illness is alleviated through a person's free-will decisions. This may be as simple as recognizing that a person has an ulcer due to mental forms of stress. The doctor advises to begin a stress relief program or life-style change. As a result, the ulcer disappears.

One case history that I heard from another hypnotherapy trainer involved a nurse who came to the realization that a lump in her breast appeared when she said to herself, "I wish I could die...(as some of her patients had)." The body heard the unconscious self-talk and responded. When she discovered this, she saw a hypnotherapist and he reframed the effect to her by pointing out that if her thoughts caused the lump, her thoughts could also make it disappear. A couple of simple suggestions were given and the lump had disappeared by the time she went for a medical examination a day or two later. Internal originated healing involves a healing by which an individual changes something within themselves that is a key to fostering the transformation.

B) <u>External Origination</u>- All healing comes from a higher power which most refer to as "God." For example, a person is ill and as a result of prayer, a religious ceremony, or a divine intervention from God, he or she experiences a healing.

In another example, an individual contracts cancer, and as a result, he or she prays for a miracle. An angel comes in a dream and tells the person to go to a place called Warm Springs, Virginia, which has a reputation for people being healed there. The person goes, receives a miraculous healing from being prayed over by a minister at the springs, and is healed. The person was healed by a higher spiritual force that was externally originated, or from outside of himself or herself.

C) <u>Combined Origination</u>- This position indicates that an individual's awareness of his or her own internal condition and mental perceptions contributed to the cause of the problem, but also divine intervention occurred and perhaps led to an individual taking a new direction in life. This affected their perceptions of themselves and their world, so the change was internal and external at the same time. For example, an individual might claim that an angel alerted him or her to a health problem through a dream. He went to the doctor, and she said that he must go on a specific medication in order to rid himself of disease symptoms. He listened to the medical advice and was healed. Both external and internal choices contributed to healing.

Though leaning a little more toward internal origination, another example of this position can be found in Hawaii. One of the oldest religions in the world is Hawaiian Huna. The spiritual leaders, the great Kahunas, taught their people that all healing comes from the divine nature within. Because our essence is spiritual by nature, we carry a spirit within each of us that is our most powerful asset. Legend has it that in order to remind the Hawaiian people of this teaching, the great kahunas turned into stone when they died. The statues can still be visited on the island of Oahu, where many who come to touch them are reminded of this teaching and are healed.

If we look at this concept from western philosophy, we find many places in the western biblical text that point to having a part of the divine within each of us. We are supposedly created in God's image. If this is true, we have abilities that are spiritual in nature for healing other individuals. If we are part of a greater whole, then we may also illuminate our inner abilities to heal, by calling on the great illuminator. The external source illuminates our internal one, and our healing abilities are strengthened. In my opinion, this ultimately describes the philosophy behind the combined origination position.

Sometimes individuals have extreme beliefs and values that may not be beneficial for maintaining a state of peace through life's normal ups and downs. These extreme values also make it difficult for individuals to utilize all of the resources that they have available when in need of a healing. The extreme individuals described below are the minority in today's society, however they can still be found. Nonetheless, the following descriptions are important for discovering the role these variables play in either facilitating or obstructing a client's ability to heal.

Extreme Individuals/Roles in Healing

Extreme Individual One (EI#1)- claims that there is nothing more beyond the physical world, no life after death. They contend that there is no spiritual nature to human beings and that our bodies are simply biochemical machines that randomly go out of balance and need biochemical adjustments or invasive procedures (surgery) to return to normal. What we think, doesn't have much impact on our bodies, nor does a higher power's will. Our thoughts may or may not change our direction. Life is a game of chance or luck. There is no hidden or higher purpose for being ill or healing.

Extreme Individual Two (EI#2)- claims that God rules everything on this planet, particularly our bodies. When we are sick, this is God's will. If we are to get well, it is God's will and there is nothing we should do to stand in the way of this intervention, not even medicine. If we are going to get better, God will make us better. We are more like puppets without free will or choice. Both good and bad happenings are a result of God's will for us. There is nothing we can change or do about it except to get God to do something about it.

EI#1 can still be found existing in western society, though this is rapidly changing with the spread of alternative health practices, holistic and spiritual concepts in the media, and educational material. EI#2 is not too prevalent either. However, there are still individuals engrossed in some fundamental religious sects who hold this view and have been known to have conflicts with the law regarding the proper medical care for their children, when the parents choose for them to go without medical care. In the era in which we live, most individuals generally don't fall under either of the extreme categories. Instead, they are going to operate somewhere in the middle, incorporating concepts into their belief structure from both extremities. The combined origination position is the principle foundation on which the general approach in this book is based.

Differentiating between the power of suggestion and the power of an externally originated healing source is a difficult task. I generally do not separate the two in describing hypnotic phenomena, because transpersonal hypnotherapy combines both principles. It includes the spiritual component of hypnosis, while putting the hypnotherapist's personal values and beliefs aside. So we will proceed with the assumption that spirit exists and the body, mind, and spirit affect each other.

Using hypnosis and the highest intention is likened to praying the client into a powerful change process. The faith factor exists because we are spiritual beings. Because we probably carry a part of the "Great Spirit" within us (a common Native American term for "God"), we have the ability to channel the highest power source in the universe through our being and into another's. This can be summarized by quoting my Reiki Master (my wife, Dee), who taught me during my study of Reiki Therapy that, "The divine within me recognizes and greets the divine within you to promote enlightenment and peace."

Chapter 4

The Mind Process

The mind process explained in this chapter was created to better understand the main functions of the mind: how the mind perceives, stores, and retrieves information. Each of these processes works interdependently and sychronistically to support the mind's ability to create meaning of an individual's internal and external environment. Because each individual has had a wide variety of completely unique life experiences, the mind process varies from one individual to the next in the use of its perceptual filters and inner components, resulting in powerful subjective thought compilations and behavioral outcomes. In a few words, this is what makes each of us so unique. The paradigm of an individual's perception of his or her past, present, and future determines behavior, both consciously and unconsciously. A shift in the paradigm alters the entire system, which leads to the inevitability of individual change or transformation. These shifts occur as constants for the purpose of evolution within the human life cycle.

In order to better understand how the functions of the mind and its perceptual factors work together, it will be beneficial to occasionally refer to the following Mind Process Model when reading different segments of this chapter.

Mind Process Model

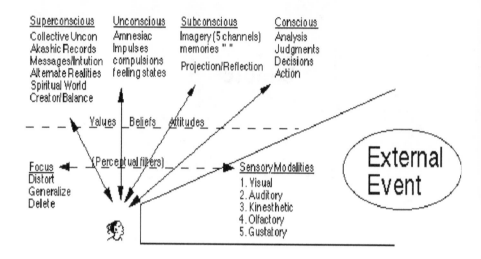

Cayce Categories of Mind

In his readings, the great modern mystic Edgar Cayce often referred to the mind using four primary categories: the conscious, subconscious, unconscious, and superconscious. We shall use these as our standards for mind function. To describe the first three categories, I will use various concepts derived from my own theories, in addition to multiple other sources in the field of clinical hypnotherapy. For defining the fourth category, the superconscious mind, I've combined some of my theories with Carl Jung's and Edgar Cayce's. Later in the book, in the chapter, The Cayce Effect, readers will be able to examine Cayce's readings where in his own words, he directly defined these categories. With this under consideration, we will proceed with the four primary categories of mind.

The Conscious Mind is known by most hypnotic research-ers as the *action part of the mind*. It chooses how to act upon the information that it is given both from the external environment and the internal environment, which triggers the imagery content derived from the other three categories of mind. Other terms used to describe the conscious mind include the "will," the "ego," the "critical sensor," and the "critical factor." Its function is to perform actions such as judging, rationalizing, deciding, and analyzing. It can only perform these functions with input from the other areas of mind; and its primary function is to make logical sense of the external world. The conscious mind cannot be detached in hypnosis, so there is a constant observational function whereby the client of hypnosis often questions what state of mind he or she is in. This questioning, or rationalizing, is a natural effect in the state of hypnosis. However, there is the need to subdue, or pacify, the conscious mind, in order for hypnosis to be therapeutically effective. Over-rationalizing will often lighten the state of hypnosis, but then deepening techniques can counteract the conscious mind's effect in this case.

Other mental functions that were discovered and utilized by the great conjoint family therapist, Virginia Satir, include generalizing, distorting, and deleting. These secondary functions of the conscious mind further help individuals create more meaning of their experience. As a result of these realizations, our logical mind will always be biased (generalization). It will always miss things we are not paying attention to (deletion); and it will always create individual logical meaning according to our past experiences (distortion). The conscious mind gives meaning to our internal and external environment through these perceptual filters.

The Subconscious Mind is referred to as the part of the mind that produces *imagery that is readily available to the conscious mind*. In daily awareness, individuals experience images in the form of five human perceptual channels: visual, auditory, kinesthetic, olfactory and gustatory. These images are selected instantaneously and automatically as the root function of the subconscious mind. How they are selected involves the purpose of the subconscious mind's selection process, which is to select the most important information involving the current subject matter at a particular time in an individual's life. It does this in the form of imagery, thereby facilitating an individual to make the most effective decisions that are possible with the resources that currently and internally exist in the mind.

The subconscious mind gets stimulated by a person concentrating on an external event, which then transposes into an internal image. This image is either a projection (of the future) or a reflection (of the past). When the subconscious chooses a future memory, it makes up a hypothetical scenario which may or may not occur at sometime in the future. Many times, a person's imagined projections do occur in some form. Nonetheless, the subconscious mind takes everything literally and personally. Everything we are exposed to becomes a subconscious experience, at least temporarily, until which point we give it something else to concentrate on.

Subconscious information may surface from the unconscious mind when a person is in a state of hypnosis. On a daily basis, primarily the information that comes forth through the subconscious is derived from memories that are easily accessible. It can also create fantasies, which are not memory material, and be actively involved as the main source of day dreaming. The subconscious mind depends on stories, or sequential imagery, in order to deepen the meaning of an experience through identification. This concept was originally discovered by Milton Erickson, who often told short stories to clients, in order to implement change. He was also known to teach hypnotherapy by simply telling stories to the class.

The Unconscious Mind is the area that produces *imagery that is generally unavailable to the conscious mind.* This area of mind often contains forgotten memories. This domain of the human mind represents the majority of our thoughts. This is where our impulses, compulsions, habits, and emotional feeling states exist which reveal root level character traits. These unconscious levels of personality are created through past experiences which convert to amnesiac memories.

The most powerful aspect of hypnosis is its ability to access root-level forms of unconscious thought and transform them. Human beings are living the majority of their lives unconsciously, or on automatic pilot. They simply take for granted that they are who and what they are, responding to life without the awareness that we are simply programmed by our unconscious mind. This dimension of mind is the domain of the emotions, which are created from experiences. From these, emotions are then stored in the great files of the unconscious mind and exist below our conscious awareness.

Many clients enter a hypnotherapist's office claiming, "I don't know why I feel this way." Often, they experience great relief from a hypnotherapy session's ability to affect and transform unconscious root-level programming, which exists as the cause of the problem. This area of mind is usually changed permanently with hypnosis. This is the primary advantage of hypnotherapy, when compared to other forms of treatment.

The Superconscious Mind is the area of mind that represents both mass consciousness and spiritual influences, or intuitive insights. It is the area that can be referred to as the aspect of mind that is the link between the unconscious process and the spirit world. Cayce referred to the superconscious as the area of mind that connects us to the akashic records. These records hold information reflecting all forms of human thought and experiences that have existed, exist now, and are likely to exist in the future. It is here that the minds of humans, angels, and other spiritual entities may transfer information to one another. In my opinion, Carl Jung referred to this same area of mind as the collective unconscious.

The superconscious mind connects us to intuition, or information about other people, places, and things. The superconscious is the least dense, or least physical, and most encompassing, whereas the conscious mind is the most dense, or most physical, and lies at the other end of the grid of human consciousness. Provided we've opened a pathway, through practicing altered states of consciousness, the superconscious mind gives us spiritual insights from the nonphysical dimensions of thought. It is for this reason that transpersonal hypnotherapy remains an expansive clinical practice. When a hypnotherapist includes the images that come to a client from the superconscious mind, he or she is practicing transpersonal hypnotherapy.

The superconscious adds a dimension that was at one time considered unimportant to the practice of hypnotherapy, and therefore not included in earlier writings on the subject. Today, most hypnotherapists have taken the next step of clinical hypnotherapy toward transpersonalism. This is because of public demand for holistic arts that include more of the whole being. Public demand comes from an evolution in the collective unconscious. For this reason, it is best to include a client's superconscious experience's in his or her sessions, when it is active.

For example, let's say Jack came into my office because he had a fear of driving, stemming from nightmares. Am I to assume that we should change Jack's unconscious programming by giving him suggestions for successful driving, or should I take into consideration that spiritual information is coming through from his superconscious mind? Perhaps Jack's reoccurring dreams indicate that Jack needs to be very cautious at intersections in the future. If Jack's dream is a warning, and he heeds the warning, he will avoid an accident. Therefore, recognizing this area of mind with all of its possible implications brings about a whole new dimension to the clinical aspects of practicing hypnotherapy. (In this regard, Carl Jung was the first to introduce intuition as an important variable in a client's therapy.)

So, does a hypnotherapist help Jack remove his fear of driving or utilize it in order to bring about a reasonable caution for avoiding an accident or a possible destiny? It appears that the vastness of possibilities that the superconscious represents brings about uncertainty for the hypnotherapist, unless they remain client centered and work within the belief system of the client. By taking this approach, the hypnotherapist is letting the client define his or her own experiences, and then synchronizing the methods with the information that is revealed during the sessions.

Another example of utilizing the superconscious would involve an individual's ability to be contacted by his or her angels. Let's say that our client is hearing an angel's voice that is being helpful to him or her. This voice would be coming from the superconscious, passing through the unconscious, and then manifesting in a client's awareness through his or her subconscious auditory channel of perception. If the hypnotherapist values this information, the hypnotherapist can utilize it in the hypnotherapy session. Hypothetically, the hypnotherapist can actually recreate the auditory messages by putting the client under hypnosis and directly accessing the superconscious dimensional reality of the client that contains the angel. (This will be discussed further in the chapter on transformational models.)

On one end of the grid, our superconscious mind offers us spiritual information about ourselves and other dimensional realities, (provided altered states of consciousness (ASCs) have opened up the boundaries between the four primary categories of mind). These pathways may be created from practicing a form of altered states of consciousness on a regular basis, (self-hypnosis, meditation, etc.), or they may be created from one hetero-hypnosis session, provided it was to a deep enough level.

The following Iceberg Model illustrates how the subconscious and unconscious, together with the superconscious, are an ocean of thought. The mind is non-local, or in other words contains thoughts and experiences from within our character, and for many, it also provides information that originates from outside of ourselves. The conscious mind is the tip of the iceberg. Our conscious mind resonates a very limited awareness level in a normal waking state, or normal state of consciousness (NSC). The purpose of this limitation is to have separate, individually unique learning experiences. The majority of our personality stems from our unconscious mind, and the superconscious that contains our alternate existence.

☞

Iceberg Model

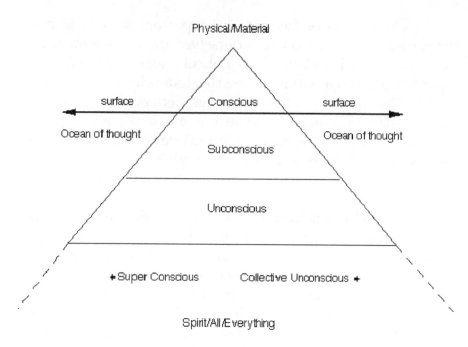

Perceptual Factors

Two very important factors of the mind that exist within each individual and serve to integrate all four categories of the mind include sensory modalities and hemispheric dominance. These variables are at the roots of perception. Of the five senses that make up perception, the senses individuals use to perceive their internal and external world most often defines a characteristic of their personality known as sensory dominance. In addition, right brain and left brain dominance also plays a role in how the sensory dominances are individually utilized.

The Five Sensory Modalities

The Five Senses are how we perceive our internal and our external world. These include the visual, auditory, kinesthetic, olfactory, and gustatory perceptual channels. These filters of perception are how we perceive and process internal and external stimuli, or information. All of the imagery that flows to our conscious mind, from our subconscious, unconscious, and superconscious areas of mind, must be sent through these five perceptual channels. Our mind utilizes these to perceive and store environmental stimuli.

1) Visual- The visual channel allows us to see our environment and store images, or representations thereof, in the mind as pictures and movies. These may surface in the mind as still pictures, color, black and white, or moving pictures.

2) Auditory- This channel generally perceives, stores, and reproduces sounds. It also provides inner conversations with ourselves known as self-talk.

3) Kinesthetic- This channel processes emotional and tactile experiences, feelings and touch. Perceptions of this kind are often channeled through, or lodged in, the physical body.

4) Olfactory- This channel allows us to perceive and store smelling experiences of the nose. Some research suggests a direct link between the sense of smell and the triggering of memories.

5) Gustatory- This channel allows us to perceive and store tasting experiences. Though less prevalent in hypnosis sessions, when gustatory experiences are present, they may be vivid.

Research shows that individuals generally show dominance in one or two primary sensory modalities. Visually dominant people will process their internal and external environment with more pictures and movies. In relation to hypnosis, the visually dominant person will *see* more of the visual portions of a hypnotherapist's suggestions, as well as memories in hypnotic regression. Likewise, an auditory person will *hear* more of the things suggested or remembered. The kinesthetic person will *feel* more of the hypnotic suggestions and memories as they enter into his or her mind. Tests are available that indicate which sensory modalities individuals use most often for learning. These tests include variables such as the visually dominant person being attracted to art, while the auditory dominant individual may be more attracted to music. The kinesthetic dominant person may often make decisions based on how they feel about certain situations.

Research also shows[7] that individuals may practice exercises that can facilitate their becoming more visual. One such exercise is glancing at a bulletin board advertisement, and then looking elsewhere while trying to remember its visual content. Although I cannot find any research for improving the other primary sensory modality systems, I am willing to make the assumption that a similar practice with sounds and feelings also probably increases clarity in these channels. A common generalization heard in the field of hypnotherapy is that it is best that individuals achieve a balance between all of the sensory modalities. Supposedly, this allows an individual to effectively be more versatile in a wider variety of circumstances. However, Dominance occurs as a result of an individual's need for a greater efficiency for performing specific tasks. Because of this, how and why these dominances form is determined by an individual's roles, or patterns of behavior, in their current life relationships and situations, such as a person's marital or career choice (i.e. a right brain dominant partner with a left brain dominant partner).

On a wider scale, most government operated education systems are designed for the visually dominant learner, although this is probably unintentional. Approximately 75% of the American population is visually dominant, so this system is effective for most of the people in the United States. Because of these factors, students in the public schools system that are more auditory or kinesthetic will not test as high as the visual ones, even though they are just as intelligent and capable. For those that are more auditory dominant, or particularly kinesthetic dominant, alternative education, such as home schooling, may be a more effective alternative. It is particularly disheartening to see a child, who is a kinesthetic learner, struggling with a low self esteem, because he or she is obtaining lower grades in the current lopsided public system. An educational system where teaching skills would include the three learning styles would increase students' memory and comprehension. In addition, including the practice of altered states as part of the daily regime would increase creativity, which would enhance critical reasoning capabilities. This is probably the wave of the future. We will be using altered states of consciousness in the educational system when society recognizes the value of such an innovative approach.

Mind, Brain, and Hemispheric Dominance

Brain is the physical aspect of a person's mental capacity, while *mind* refers to the metaphysical or nonphysical aspect. While brain can be found in the body as a physical member, mind is assumed to be the higher more holographic component of thought. It is the higher-self component that exists both within and above the body, similar to an observer looking down on the brain's process of thought. Some believe mind is the spiritual component of our brain that is connected to a higher power or creative source.

Left brain functioning involves the conscious mind's functions of rationalizing, analyzing, judging, and logical decisions. Right brain activity involves the use of impressions, imagery, and imagination. The mind process model may be divided into right and left brain counterparts by drawing a vertical line between the conscious mind, or left brain functions, and the subconscious, unconscious, and superconscious dimensions of mind, which are considered to be right brain functions.

The extreme right brain dominant person looks at a forest and describes smelling the trees, the beautiful sun light, and the feeling of the pine needles, while the extreme left brain dominant person looks at the same forest and describes the process of photosynthesis and the food chain. It is important to understand, however, that each of these individuals, regardless of how dominant, use both hemispheres of their brains in order to be functional. Readers may find it helpful to refer to the mind process model at the beginning of this chapter to understand more fully the right brain/left brain hemispheric functioning divisions and operations relative to other mental activities within the mind.

Research shows that hypnosis is generally a right brain activity. Right brain activities involve the process of identifying with impressions or images. All of the applied altered states of consciousness (AASCs) that are listed in chapter one, may be classified as right brain dominant activities. It is the right brain dominant individuals that experience the subconscious, unconscious, and superconscious dimensions of mind in a more vivid and compelling fashion, both in and out of the altered state. Right brain dominant individuals also generally undergo hypnosis more quickly, and they experience deeper levels of trance than those that are left brain dominant. Individuals who are right brain dominant tend to be in occupations such as factory worker, artist, hypnotherapist, minister, yoga instructor, interior designer, architect, musician, writer, and more.

Left brain dominant individuals can undergo hypnosis well, but they have more conscious-mind chatter during the process. It is this chatter that needs to be managed properly in order for a client to learn to successfully enter and maintain a state of hypnosis. When it comes to accomplishing tasks, left brain dominant individuals generally have a knack for "making things happen." They are characterized as more organized, logical, and systematic. Occupations in which left brain dominant individuals can generally be found include: computer programmer, scientist, medical doctor, accountant, military officer, auditor, and more.

All individuals have some combination of right brain and left brain functioning, but when tested with dominance exams, we usually indicate dominance in one hemisphere or the other. The left brain dominant individual can become more right brain dominant, if he or she practices more altered states of consciousness, such as self-hypnosis or meditation. In addition, an individual may consider engaging in more right brain activities, such as playing music or creating art. As a result, hypnosis and other altered states of consciousness will become easier and more enjoyable. Likewise, right brain dominant individuals may become more left brain dominant by using their logical mind more often, such as trying to focus on how things function from a systematic perspective. Studying systems or mechanical concepts help to develop the left brain.

Many individuals who are highly dominant in either the left or right hemisphere unconsciously maintain friendships, or spousal relationships, with somebody having the opposite dominance. This also happens for the purpose of achieving a productive balance in business by choosing partners or coworkers with an opposite dominance from our own. This is why we see the musician, for example, who is often right brain dominant, with the business manager, who is often left brain dominant. In another case, we may notice one spouse engrossed in seeking and experiencing spiritual experiences, while the other spouse tends to analyze these experiences to make them more logical for both parties. Therefore, a balance exists to create a more effective team for approaching societies challenges, and each person's personality becomes more rounded in the union over time.

Three Primary Components of Values

The three primary components that exist within a person's valuation process, or what we commonly refer to as "values," include attitudes, beliefs, and values—values having two subcategories: those being clusters of value around specific subject matters, and those core values which are more fixed. Each component operates slightly different within the inner self, depending on a person's sociobiographical influences (family, upbringing), and his or her societal influences, (socioeconomic, culture, etc.).

Attitudes change from day to day. People commonly associate them with moods. Those that have more frequent or more dramatic attitude shifts are often referred to as "moody." "Level headed" individuals generally are not as easily excitable and have more stable moods or attitudes. Moods are often labeled "good" or "bad," and are more of an internal gauge for each individual. This gauge allows people to judge their environmental conditions as being either painful or pleasurable. The "Pain-Pleasure Principle" was made popular through Tony Robbins' book, *Unlimited Power*, which popularized Neurolinguistic Programming (NLP) and altered states of consciousness with the general public. He said that people are either motivated away from pain or toward pleasure. Many of Tony Robbins' seminars teach people how to accomplish the dissolution of their fears, or change their attitudes, by rehearsing repetitive affirmations and then fire walking by the end of the night. Those with mental, physical, or spiritual limitations often shed them through the attitude adjustments which often occur during these seminars.

At a time when they were most popular, I was invited to attend one of these seminars, in the mid 1990s, in Washington,

DC. There were approximately 13 large fires and well over 1000 people who all "walked the fire" that night. Attitudes affect beliefs, which lie at the root of attitudes. Beliefs affect attitudes and visa versa. This is how people can literally walk on fire without getting burned, and metaphorically do so in many of their life's scenarios thereafter.

Attitude change is the area that suggestive therapy affects most often and most easily. In fact, I state to my clients that, in addition to daily relaxation, the biggest benefit of using hypnotherapy to change a habit is attitude shifts. They simply will not feel like _____ing anymore; they will focus on other things instead. Attitudes are key factors to making substantial changes in life, and being at peace more often in the process.

Beliefs are primarily made up of logic from significant life experiences, which eventually become internal representations of those events. As new significant experiences occur from year to year, people's belief structures change. As a result, their logical explanation of exactly what they believe also transforms. In fact, if an individual is engaged in a conversation describing his or her beliefs to another person, and the listener repetitively asks, "Why? Why do you believe that?," the speaker will eventually describe significant life experiences from within his or her memory. However, this form of questioning may be seen as an interrogation, if it is not done with compassion. It is important for a transpersonal hypnotherapist to allow all belief structures to exist, and to recognize that these logical explanations of a person's experiences are necessary for his or her spirit to have entered into the material world, embraced an individualized path through time, and thereby have taught and learned concepts in his or her own unique, destined fashion.

Each belief has clusters of attitudes surrounding it. Beliefs also represent the logic behind an individual's core values; therefore, each core value has clusters of beliefs surrounding it. Often, extreme beliefs are a result of core values, or a person's spiritual experiences. Therefore, beliefs can be an important means of understanding a clients' perceptions about themselves and their world.

If clients' beliefs are working well for them, then there is no need to question or change them. If they are not facilitating clients in making productive changes, or reaching a higher level of peace in their lives, it may be time to question the experiences that created those beliefs and transform them by way of hypnotherapeutic intervention. This is frequently the case with hypnotherapy clients. Most change that results from hypnotherapy, or any therapy, is derived from changing beliefs.

Values are similar to beliefs in that they can be driven by memories, but the energy behind a value is much stronger. A value gives a person's beliefs purpose and movement toward and away from certain concepts. Negative values correlate with people, places, or things, and have pain associated with them, while positive values have pleasurable associations. Values determine the outcome of behavior and therefore are at the root of motivation.

When values are in conflict, movement becomes stagnant. In other words, it leads to indecision. For example, let's say that Jill has a desire for a romantic relationship, but because she has had one or two that were very painful in the past, she avoids them completely. As a result, it is best to help Jill transform her negative values. When negative values are transformed, individuals are able to set positive goals for themselves and achieve them.

Core Values are deeper than normal values. They answer the question, "Why am I alive?" They put an individual into a deep energetic, or unconsciously-driven state of motivation. Core values are often at the root of a person's spirituality. Significant belief clusters surround core values and indicate the purpose of being alive in human existence. The more positive an individual's core values are, the higher his or her energy level is when approaching tasks. When core values are in conflict, suicidal thoughts and/or major life changes may occur. Often, the result of resolving relative inner conflicts is a complete revamping of a person's relationships, career, and purpose in life.

When a client's therapeutic goal involves spiritual growth, such as meeting with spirit guides or regressing into past-lives, etc., the client may open up the core of his or her being, which often leads to reconsidering his or her true nature and finding greater purpose within human life. This is successful in the long term only if a transpersonal hypnotherapist stays client centered. Converting a client to a therapist's deepest core values, by promoting spiritual beliefs, is generally unsuccessful in the long-term, and often results in the client terminating therapy. This is because each individual has unique experiences, and if those significant life experiences do not match those of the therapist, or the leader of another religion or philosophy, values or beliefs will be in conflict at some point in time. This is simply because there will be a lack of experience to support it.

To summarize, values are pertinent to therapeutic change. Lighter structure values such as pain-pleasure principles are key for changing things like habits, while deeper structure values, such as the purpose for being alive in a human body, are at the deeper roots of a person's energetic or unconscious levels of motivation.

There are several types of questionnaires available for students of hypnotherapy that will help them discover a person's brain dominance and sensory modality dominance. By this time, readers should have some ability to create assumptions about the mind processes of both themselves and their clients. These factors are of most importance to hypnotherapists, because they determine how clients will experience hypnosis. Once these are studied, experienced, and understood, the result is increased rapport and the achievement of therapeutic goals. Some hypnotherapists have personality profiling tests that are given to their clients before the first session. Others simply observe and ask pertinent questions regarding the client's experiences under hypnosis, in order to make logical deductions concerning perceptual dominances. Either way, these are important factors for increasing success in a clinical hypnotherapy practice.

Chapter 5

Primary Directives of the Unconscious Mind

The domain of the rather abstract unconscious mind primarily involves metaphorical, involuntary thought patterns. Its more concrete partner is the subconscious mind, but because the subconscious is very similar in function, the terms "subconscious" and "unconscious" are often used interchangeably by hypnotherapists. The unconscious domain of mind involves certain purposes, or directives. These *Prime Directives* of the unconscious mind include:

Storing and Organizing Memories
Storing and Operating Emotions
Operating and Preserving the Physical Body
Valuing Pain and Pleasure Experiences
Experiencing and Replicating the World Metaphorically
Accepting Things Literally and Personally
Maintaining Genealogical Instincts
Creating and Maintaining Least-Effort Patterns
Co-creating the Future Through Imagination
Providing Doorways to Spiritual Awareness
<u>Storing and Organizing Memories:</u> All unconscious and sub-

conscious information is formulated from memories. Individuals store each experience they have through the conscious mind's filters of perception which include: generalization; deletion; and distortion. Out of these three, generalization continues to serve as a primary interactive perceptual function for the subconscious and unconscious areas of mind. Each individual's new experience has generalizations attached to it which are derived from prior experiences, therefore, every human being is biased automatically and according to his or her past experiences. Generalizations work harmoniously with beliefs as a logical conscious mind deduction.

Thoughts, feelings, and memories often get triggered, so that each individual may mentally operate at peak efficiency in regards to each environmental situation that is encountered. The objective, by way of design, is to allow past experiences to be imagined at the most appropriate time to allow each individual to respond with the most appropriate action. The data available to an individual's awareness through the subconscious mind and the unconscious mind is limited to the experiences that are programmed into them, unless a hypnotherapist includes the transpersonal aspects of the superconscious mind, or spiritual thoughts. The unconscious mind absorbs new information in every moment, which is why adults are more proficient than children in responding to their environment. They simply have had more experiences stored in their unconscious minds to act upon.

Although the intention of these areas of mind is to facilitate efficiency, there are times when individuals have subconscious memories or impulses that disturb them. This process is referred to as *stress rehearsal* and is an archetypal process for all humans. With each rehearsal, the memory changes until it is imagined with less discomfort. Often the subconscious will recycle these until they are resolved. The stressful memories range from childhood and before to that which has transpired only moments ago. Resolution often comes when new thoughts intervene during a person's repetition of a stressful memory.

Storing and organizing memories occurs in many various ways, but rehearsal is one of its primary functions. Resolution and creating understanding is this directives primary purpose.

<u>Storing and Operating Emotions:</u> Emotions are generally cre-

ated from significant life experiences which are then stored meta-phorically as memories, either subconsciously or unconsciously. Those emotions that are stored in the unconscious realm of mind are the most powerful, as their origins, in the form of memories, are unconscious, so they surface in the form of impulses and compulsions. The decision to behave one way or another is based on how a person feels about specific subject matters. Emotions are at the root of behavior. They are the driving force for making decisions. When emotions are in operation, individuals are either driven toward pleasure or away from pain. Therefore, emotions determine a person's motivation level.

Emotions also interface with the conscious process of generalization. Emotion is usually attached to memories when subconsciously recalled by individuals. Pleasurable memories are triggered by a pleasant experience in the environment, while painful memories are often triggered by painful experiences. The role of the subconscious mind is to bring forth the emotion that fits the current experience. Emotions often surface subconsciously with their memory counterparts on a daily level. From time to time, they also surface without a subconscious memory, indicating their memory counterparts remain unconscious. Unfortunately, the emotion retrieved is not always the most appropriate one for an individual's environment, so a conscious decision is made that a person needs to either curb his or her emotional response or create a new one. It is with these un-rooted emotions that hypnotherapy uniquely benefits individuals the most.

Clients who have unpleasant unconsciously driven emo-tions will often tell me, "I don't know why I feel this way," and it is usually forgotten, unconscious memories that are causing the problem. Many clients of this type begin to doubt their own ability to be rational, and sometimes resort to addictions or psychotropic medications, when free floating anxiety seems to be at its peak. By bringing the root-causative memories for these emotions to light, either in the interview process for suggestive therapy, or under hypnotic regression, the client is often freed from his or her problematic emotions. These emotions may be the cause of a wide range of problems in the client's relationships and situations.

The unconscious mind utilizes emotions for facilitating a

person's effectiveness in life. Emotions are necessary to gauge experiences but, when they are out of balance, they often lead to disharmony within the self, and within the surrounding environment.

Operating and Preserving the Physical Body: The unconscious mind assists in operating and preserving the body with thoughts and emotions. This can be documented neurologically through that which neuroscientists refer to as gray matter in the brain. The autonomic nervous system operates various areas of the body, such as the heart, immune system, respiration, and more. Thoughts and feelings are stored in the body. Kinesiologists often demonstrate the effect of thought on the body by performing muscle testing. With positive thoughts, the muscles are stronger when a person is asked to resist downward pressure on the arm. With negative thoughts, a person's muscles are shown to become weaker.

Stage hypnotists can demonstrate full-body catalepsy by having a hypnotized subject imagine that she is "stiff as a board," as it is illustrated below. Then, they lay the person's body across two chairs, demonstrating an unusual amount of strength to stay horizontal. Therefore, it may be theorized that what people say to themselves and hear in their environment directly affects their bodies.

Full-Body Catalepsy

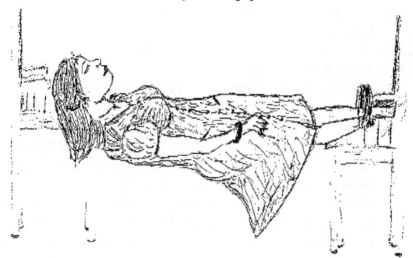

To further understand the relationship between the mind and the body, we could glance at the work of Dr. Bruce Lipton. Lipton is a mind-body researcher, with degrees in neuroscience from Stanford and the University of Virginia, who speaks regularly at various conventions and medical colleges. He has proven the body's cellular structure to be holographic. In other words, thoughts have been shown to affect every cell in the body. One of the studies he cites in his research involves military subjects who view a movie with emotional content, while their skin cells are measured for galvanic skin response. A piece of skin is measured at the same time five hundred miles away. Both skin samples show the same response. This and other forms of research prove that every cell of the body responds to thought, and the unconscious mind affects every cell holographically.

He also found that the body's immune response can double with a strong emotion associated with a trauma to body tissues, such as a sliver in the skin. Thus, in fact, hyper-immune problems may be curbed with proper emotional reactions to stress. This may help explain why people can walk on 1400 degree coals, without getting burned and blistering—or stimulating white blood cells to congregate. The emotional component may be the key.

Conversely, with high amounts of stress, it appears that the immune system can lose its ability to destroy foreign cells, like cancer, which regularly enter a person's body. Change can be the most stressful factor in a person's life. Research shows that many adults who contract cancer had experienced a major loss, such as the death of a loved one, within a two year period[8]. Hypnotherapy can be a valuable intervention for resolving forms of grief or loss more quickly, before this condition has a chance to deplete the body. In addition, according to Bernie Siegel, M.D., imagery and hypnosis can help eliminate cancer cells after they have become a problem.

Self-hypnosis and hypnotherapy can help more positive thoughts enter into the mind and reduce stress by creating more positive responses to life's situations. Hypnosis serves as a bridge between the mind and body, and one primary purpose of the unconscious mind is to assist in the operation and preservation of the body.

Experiencing and Replicating the World Metaphorically: Our thoughts are not an objective, concrete replication of our environmental experiences, as most people think they are. Instead, they are internal representations in the form of metaphors or symbols. These represent our external experiences. Thoughts are subjective meanings for the past, present and future realities. All thought, therefore, is subjective, using imagination; and memories are metaphors for experiences, which can change, at least to some degree, over time.

Imagination is not pretend, false, or unreal. In fact, it is the determining factor for our concept of reality. The word imagination is defined in Webster's Dictionary as "The production of imagery." Whether or not a memory is accurate depends on several biological, social, and psychological factors. Psychologically, imagination is the pathway to retrieving memories both in a normal and altered state of consciousness.

Imagination, therefore, is the foundation for our reality. Through a process of vivification, it involves thoughts and experiences that we automatically and unconsciously give credence to.

Because each individual creates a form of self-identity from these metaphorical representations, a great importance is generally placed on the ability to have accurate memory. When a person's memories are changed under hypnosis, such as in hypnotic regression, it generally leads to a transformation. Suggestive therapy also shifts memories, but more indirectly. In addition, memories can change by themselves, so this leads a person to theorize that our identity is always evolving and time is simply nothing more than a perception.

Some would even refer to time as an illusion, since the only place where time can be accessed is within the self. In other words, the concepts of past, present, and future are only in the mind, and the now is where we draw these perceptions from. Another way to look at it is that each mind is a universe of time, and hypnosis is the time machine, or vehicle, which allows people to access time and therefore produce paradigm shifts. Once a memory is transformed, a person's past, present, and future changes simultaneously, which is a collective conscious overlay on the external environment.

Although memories are metaphorical in nature, and therefore subjective, research shows that they often prove to be extremely accurate. Even forensic science utilizes hypnosis extensively based on its proven ability to help witnesses recall more details to crimes. Because our unconscious mind stores about 2000 bits of information per second, sometimes investigators extract details out of a hypnotized subject's peripheral vision, in order to track down assailants. Hypnotic research utilizing memories proves that these metaphors can certainly prove to be accurate.

<u>Accepting Things Literally and Personally</u>: The subconscious and unconscious minds do *not process negatives* under hypnosis. Even in the waking state, when an individual suggests a sentence with a negative in it, a person's subconscious mind will first imagine every word, before it cancels out the idea to create an opposite one. In our left brain dominant society, we may refer to this common behavior as the process of elimination. However, the subconscious mind is like a child's mind. It hears everything on a very simple level. If we tell a very young child, "Don't spill that milk," the next thing that often happens is the spilling of the milk. The child imagined spilling the milk and did not take the second mental step of imagining how not to spill the milk, since a child's subconscious mind is more active than that of an adult's.

Nonetheless, adults are also affected by "negative people" or "positive people." We can see a person's facial expression change when we mention both pleasant and unpleasant concepts, which are imagined unconsciously, automatically and unconditionally.

The subconscious mind takes everything personally, particularly in hypnosis. Therefore, it is advisable that hypnotherapists always remain aware of the literal value of their suggestions. Every word creates meaning in the subconscious and unconscious realms of mind. These areas of mind do not detect negatives the way the conscious mind does, so outcome-based hypnotic suggestions are generally more effective when using hypnosis to influence peoples' behaviors.

Maintaining Genealogical Instincts: Unconscious thought processes include the thoughts and behaviors of our ancestors. The most valued experiences, which are those geared toward survival, are genetically passed on to our unconscious minds and operate in the form of impulses. It may even be termed as genetic memory. The most common function of these memories is the *fight or flight response*. This response to stressful situations allows us to fight an oncoming threat, or flee from it.

Hypothetically, when we were cavemen and were threatened with a surprise attack, we needed to be able to think fast and respond with effectively fleeing or fighting. Most often these episodes occurred while in the relaxing surroundings of the wilderness, and we were taken by surprise. Our bodies thereby learned to respond to life or death situations by providing a burst of energy.

The "stress response" and the "relaxation response" were terms created by Herbert Benson, MD, while performing extensive research into our genealogical stress factors. According to Dr. Benson, the *stress response* stems from the fight or flight response; it is characterized by increased respiration, increased heart rate, increased metabolism, sweaty palms, dry mouth, beta brain waves, and the secretion of adrenaline into the blood stream. The *relaxation response* represents the opposite. It is characterized by lowered respiration, lowered heart rate, lowered metabolism, a decrease in blood pressure, and predominant alpha brain waves.

Although the stress response can serve a purpose, it gets triggered too frequently, due to the increased amount of environmental stimuli within our society. As a result, situations are often unconsciously perceived as a threat, or life or death situation, which increases stress and its resulting health risks. Because of this, in order to counteract stress, it becomes necessary to regularly practice altered state of consciousness, self-hypnosis being the most efficient and effective.

Other genetic programs include eating, sleeping, reproduction, glandular function—such as salivating, and more. The unconscious mind contains more genealogical instincts than can be listed, and many are useful for being a more effective human being.

Creating and Maintaining Least-Effort Habit Patterns: It has often been said that human beings are "creatures of habit." All patterns, or habits, enhance an individual's abilities for learning new information. Once a habit is established in the subconscious mind, an individual may comfortably run the pattern with very little effort and then focus on new, more important tasks. Triggers in the environment automatically and unconsciously set off patterns. Most would agree that patterns relieve stress, unless they cause bad side effects, such as health problems. In those cases, a habit tends to cause more stress than it relieves, so the individual attempts to eradicate it. However, it can be difficult to create a new habit with the motivations of health and prosperity, because these are consciously weighed against an individual's immediate gratifications. These old, familiar unhealthy habits, or short term stress relievers, have been regularly relied upon, in some cases, for many years. Therefore habits, which are rooted in the unconscious mind, are most effectively transformed with hypnosis—which is an intervention that primarily involves the domain of the unconscious mind.

Once a pattern is installed in the unconscious mind, the conscious mind can concentrate on other things. In essence, the mind is free to compile learnings. Without patterns, each individual would be in disarray, because there would be nothing but innate, animalistic instincts to draw upon to master our daily tasks. More than genetic programming is necessary to be a productive human being that is on a higher path.

Experiential learning is a result of a higher intention for learning and evolution; and the unconscious mind is the key to keeping our experiences stored and patterned.

Co-creating the Future Through Imagination: Imagination is a subconscious function. Whatever we focus on in our imagination will become a future reality in some way, shape or form. Many times during my second session interview, when my client claimed difficulty in the acceptance of the clinical suggestions given from the first session, I would ask, "Did you imagine yourself as a ____ (their goal) like I suggested?" The client's response has consistently been, "No, I couldn't imagine it." The client had the willpower to work on it, but the power of the imagination was a key ingredient that was left out of the recipe for change. The rule of thumb for creating a desired future, particularly with the use of hypnosis, is the ability to use positive goal-oriented imagination. If he or she is able to do that, the desired future will then occur in some way, shape, or form.

Clients generally get exactly what they imagined under hypnosis. Under this premise, we could theorize that our *imagination* is the recipe for our free will and the part of ourselves that serves as a blueprint for future materialization. The future is largely determined, then, on what we as individuals imagine and put our energy into, particularly with emotionally driven images. Images with these *emotional drivers* make a person's imagination manifest more quickly. If we fear, then that is what manifests; if we have positive dreams for the future, then that is what manifests. Hypnosis amplifies imagination. Under hypnosis, we can step into and live the desired future before we get there. Because of the ability of hypnosis to vivify imagination, imagination is more powerful under hypnosis than in the waking state, particularly for creating desirable future outcomes.

Providing Doorways to Spiritual Awareness: There are multiple ways to "connect" to a higher power, and generally they involve the use of an altered state and a person's imagination (prayer, meditation, hypnosis, etc.). After connecting, there are many types of miraculous results that often take place. Edgar Cayce also talked about how the use of a person's "imaginative forces" leads to opening up a person's consciousness to new spiritual dimensions of awareness. In other words, imagination is the key to the unconscious mind and creating new spiritual awareness.

If we look at the concept of prayer (an altered state) in this light, we find that there is an aspect to it that involves a person's imagination. What is it in a person's prayer imagination, unconsciously, that creates the "request" part of the equation to get spiritual graces? Certainly, there is enough research floating around out there in the field of holistic health that proves that prayer gets results, and there must be something particular to the altered state that gives the unconscious mind the ability to create these "door ways" to spiritual awareness and connectedness.

Hypnosis is another doorway to expand a person's spiritual awareness. Utilizing it non-directively, an individual may spontaneously experience angels, past-lives, plus greater awareness of self and others. This level of awareness, for most people, is generally not present when in a normal everyday state of consciousness.

Transpersonal hypnotherapists recognize and involve the client's higher power influences in their approach; and often the way by which these influences are experienced by clients varies widely. Therefore, information people share about the channels with which they are making the spiritual connection (meditation, prayer, psychics, hypnosis, etc.) needs to be handled with the utmost honor and respect, in order for sessions to be effective on a higher and more powerful level.

Upon request, I've helped my clients recognize their own unique relationship to the God source and help them explore new ways to develop it. Using self-hypnosis to meditate on a white light, and sometimes a spirit-guide—or angel, is one way to help a client make a spiritual connection. Though meditation is almost universally accepted, there are many other ways that are worth exploring in which a transpersonal hypnotherapist may assist clients in creating this important link to spirit.

In my many years of clinical work in psychological, psychiatric, and personal growth settings, I've focused on loving and accepting my clients where they are at that point in their evolution. In turn, they love who and what they are more, which is an important factor in healing, making changes, and finding peace.

There are many prime directives of the unconscious mind. Their purposes are numerous, but their primary function is to stimulate human potential. It appears that all are geared toward human evolution, which means that change is inherent for the human being. We are set on a path of learning for a higher purpose, with a higher intention. Sometimes we humans catch glimpses of enlightenment when considering evolutionary concepts. Hypnotherapy, and states of self-hypnosis, can provide unique experiences for these moments of enlightenment.

Chapter 6

Misconceptions of Hypnosis

Misconceptions have both plagued the profession of hypnosis, and rewarded it. In the past, it has either been an obstacle for people to try hypnosis or the cause of a burning interest. This primarily depends on the perceptions of the interested party. For those who believe it is too dangerous or risky, misconceptions have prevented them from enjoying the benefits it has to offer. For those who believe that hypnosis can magically or radically alter their mind, or their personality traits, misconceptions have facilitated their trying hypnosis.

Misconceptions of hypnosis commonly include:

1) Weak-minded or unintelligent people make better subjects.
2) The hypnotherapist should have an authoritarian approach.
3) Some people may not be able to awaken from hypnosis.
4) Hypnosis causes people to lose control and reveal secrets.
5) Hypnosis has harmful effects.
6) Hypnosis is a state of sleep.
7) Hypnosis is a form of brain washing.

1) Weak-minded or unintelligent people make better subjects.

Actually, the opposite is true. The more strong-willed a client is, the better the results. This is because their concentration level in better. Once a strong-willed person sets his or her sights on something he or she wants, or wants to change, their concentration is expanded, and the commitment to achieve the desired result increases the power of the suggestions. In addition, those with higher I.Q.s have an increased ability to concentrate, so they have a greater ability to imagine the desired results. This creates a higher degree of success, because concentration is a key factor to being able to imagine suggestions.

2) The hypnotherapist should have an authoritarian approach.

The idea that a person must be a dominant hypnotist in order to be effective comes from entertainment hypnosis. *Authoritarian methods* are utilized to demonstrate to the audience the dramatic effects of suggestion. An example of authoritarian methods would be to say, "Sleep," while reaching out and closing a person's eyelids with the wave of the hand. In stage hypnosis, it appears that the subjects are being commanded to do ridiculous acts, when in fact the hypnotist is just putting on a show. Truly, those who have volunteered to go on stage and act silly are usually under a deep state of hypnosis, and likely the most susceptible to the altered state. However, these individuals are also selected to stay on the stage throughout the show, because they are the most motivated to go along with the humorous suggestions, or they would not have volunteered in the first place. During the show, generally there are some subjects who try to prove that they are not under hypnosis by denying the suggestions. These subjects are told to leave the stage and go sit down in the audience.

For the purpose of private practice, it is strongly advisable for an individual to use the *permissive approach*, because people generally are put off by the less compassionate aspects of the authoritarian approach, when it comes to working with personal problems. In general, people don't like to be told what to do. In the permissive approach, the client is gradually and gently coaxed into a pleasant state of hypnosis and the use of suggestion is done in a very collaborative fashion.

3) Some people may not be able to awaken from hypnosis.

As a general rule, people awaken from hypnosis rather easily. The ego cannot be detached under hypnosis, so there is a subtle awareness at all times within clients that they are under a relaxed state of mind in a location in which they are familiar. There are those that believe hypnosis can be likened to an out-of-body experience, however, or in other words, the soul leaves the body.

This probably happened to Edgar Cayce when a sheet of paper was passed over his head during a reading. I believe that the particular altered state that Mr. Cayce entered into for performing readings was somnambulistic hypnosis, but of a rare delta level. In other words, even though Cayce was never hooked up to an electroencephalograph for measuring his brain waves, it is quite possible that he was in delta brain waves. Delta is generally impossible to reach for the majority of the population, except in some cases of well practiced yogis. It may be hypothesized that the cord, which some yogis describe when leaving their body, may have been severed temporarily during the session that resulted in Cayce staying in the hypnotic state for over twenty-four hours. Perhaps Cayce's soul consciousness frequently left his body, while still being attached by the silver cord, in order to explore other realms of consciousness (for more information, see the chapter, The Cayce Effect).

At this point, it is important to note that I have never encountered anything of the sort with the thousands of hypnotized individuals that I've worked with over several years of private practice. Because of this, I believe that all individuals may exit hypnosis at any time. Sometimes some individuals resist awakening or may have slipped out of hypnosis and into sleep; and these individuals must be coaxed out of trance, in order to end the session within a predetermined period of time. (For more information regarding resisting awakening, refer to the chapter, Induction and Awakening Procedures).

4) Hypnosis causes people to lose control and reveal secrets.

Hypnosis is a state of relaxation, so people under hypnosis do tend to divulge more information than they would in a normal waking state. Yet, this would be seen by most clinicians as a major benefit. This is an effect that every human being experiences simply by being relaxed. With hypnosis, resistances which are normally present during the waking state are reduced. Not only is this a major credit to hypnosis, but in many cases a primary strength over other forms of therapy. Although some traditional therapists have been known to argue that hypnosis reduces a person's resistances too quickly, there is no real danger, because deep secrets will not be divulged unless a client wants to express them. Again, hypnosis does not detach the ego, or the will, so the normal state of homeostasis that an individual commonly maintains in the waking state will be present. Hypnosis does not cause a loss of control.

<u>5) Hypnosis has harmful effects.</u>

The effect of hypnosis has never been known to be harmful to anyone. Primary effects from a state of hypnosis that have been known to occur include: relaxation, stress reduction, attitude adjustment, increased awareness, and intuition. These have been clinically proven through many sources. The relaxation effect can last approximately twenty four hours. For this reason, it is beneficial for an individual to do self-hypnosis, or listen to a self-hypnosis tape once a day, particularly when attempting to change a habit. It simply takes the stress out of making the change, so it is easier to accomplish.

In addition, people have been known to become more intuitive by practicing altered states. The deeper the state of hypnosis achieved, generally, the clearer the pathway for intuitive images to manifest. Sometimes, if an individual wants to maintain the effect of receiving intuitive images, he or she must undergo a deep state of hypnosis provided by another hypnotherapist every once in a while. This is generally because a deeper state of hypnosis is experienced through hetero-hypnosis than that which may be achieved through self-hypnosis. However, becoming proficient at self-hypnosis is another way to expand self awareness, as we shall see in the chapter on self-hypnosis when this state progresses to the stages of transcendental meditation.

6) Hypnosis is a state of sleep.

Hypnosis is a state of mind which lies *between awake and asleep*. Sleep is where the conscious mind detaches and becomes one with our unconscious mind, and the two flow together. Hypnosis is where we still have the ego, or the conscious mind, present in the current awareness, while there is a production of subconscious and unconscious imagery. Through the altered state, the unconscious mind transfers information to the conscious mind, so we can be aware of subconscious and unconscious thoughts. Sleep is whereby the unconscious and conscious minds become one.

If I ask a hypnotized client, who has fallen asleep, to have a memory, he or she would simply continue to snore, not hearing me at all. However, if I ask a hypnotized client who has fallen asleep to awaken when I count from five back to one, he or she is likely to awaken at the number one. This is because the sleep state began with hypnosis. This is what I call *hypnosleep*. Indeed, people are still open to suggestion during the sleep state, but hypnosis is not sleep.

So if clients ask, "Am I going to fall asleep?" I respond with the possibility that they *could* fall asleep, but that's not our goal. Our goal is hypnosis. As a result of fatigue, a client can pass out of the hypnotic state and into sleep and still receive the benefit of the hypnotic suggestions. Most clients who listen to their self-hypnosis tapes at bed time fall asleep to them, because they are naturally fatigued. Yet, they get results. I tell my clients that hypnosis is not sleep; hypnosis is a state of relaxation between awake and asleep.

7) Hypnosis is a form of brain washing.

Hypnosis is not brain washing. If it were, the ideas expressed by a hypnotist to a subject would be called "commands" rather than "suggestions." It is this misconception that scares the general public the most. When hypnosis is put to the extremes for entertainment, people may act silly, but they never commit antisocial acts, do things against their morals, values, or better judgment. They are not brain washed.

Brain washing generally consists of a combination of breaking down the conscious mind and a weak belief structure, beliefs being at the root of logic. Such tortures as sleep deprivation and dropping a steady drip of water on someone's forehead have led to the breaking down of the conscious mind. These acts reduce a person's ability to sort ideas in a rational fashion. As a result, the mind becomes susceptible to questioning reality, which often leads to the installation of a new belief structure.

In addition, there are people who have weakly organized belief structures and will seek out fanatical authority figures or groups that provide them with such structure. These personality types surrender their ego more easily than normal people do, to believe what an authority figure says is true. Cults are not using tortuous physical tactics to affect the belief structure, but more of a process I call core values manipulation. In other words, the brainwashed person in a cult is led to believe that an individual or group is led by God for a cause. This cause is believed in without question. Another example is where wars have been fought with military subjects brain washed into believing that murder leads to heaven. Kamikaze missions, for example, and other suicide bombings of our day, involve brain washing.

Hypnosis has nothing to do with the breaking down or sur-rendering of the ability to rationalize. It is a safe, pleasant process of relaxation and suggestion, automatically keeping self preserva-tion in tact. The subconscious mind can either accept or reject the suggestions given. If these are in alignment with a client's beliefs, values, and motivations that are in existence, the hypnotherapy client stands a good chance for success.

Describing Hypnotherapy to Others

The following is a list of the most frequent questions that have been asked by my clients over a number of years. It can be given to a client in the waiting room, and answer a lot of concerns be-forehand. This can facilitate the interview process so that client and hypnotherapist spend less time talking about misconceptions and more time talking about therapeutic goals.

What is Hypnotherapy?

The Most Frequent Questions:
Answered By Dr. Allen S. Chips

Question: What is hypnosis?

Answer: A state of relaxation and/or a level of concentration that the average individual reaches daily. Self-hypnosis is accomplished most often when an individual is absorbed in a TV program, experiencing repetition (highway driving), or daydreaming. "Hypnotherapy" is a form of guided relaxation using concentration where the ideas expressed (suggestions) by the therapist are generally experienced more vividly, which in turn creates a new awareness. Depending on a person's motivations, there may be a shift in attitude about specific subject matters, such as habits and stress. The only requirement for getting therapeutic results is that the person has a conscious desire to change, or in other words, is in agreement with the suggestions.

Question: Do people do things under hypnosis that are against their morals or values?

Answer: No. Hypnosis cannot detach the ego. As a general rule, if a client were given a suggestion he or she did not agree with, he or she would simply refuse, laugh at it, or awaken from hypnosis. In stage hypnosis, the volunteers are usually under the influence of alcohol and have come to the show for the purpose of relaxing, acting silly, and having a good time. Therefore, they are easily encouraged to do so. Because inhibitions are often reduced under hypnosis, the subject is more likely to experience his or her inner character traits and motivations. Yet, if an individual deems these inner character traits inappropriate, they do not reveal them. Beliefs and values continue to stay intact during any act that involves hypnosis.

Question: Can a person's memory be erased?

Answer: No. If an individual undergoing hypnosis wants to remember what happened under hypnosis, or have memories from the past, he or she will. In some cases, if the client wants to forget something, amnesia can be produced with a post-hypnotic suggestion, but it wears off as quickly as the subject wishes. However, a certified hypnotherapist can help a person transform a memory which may be causing problems. The mind contains unconscious memories which generally are responsible for our decisions, attitudes, feelings, and behaviors.

Question: Can everyone be hypnotized?

Answer: Yes, provided an individual has normal physiological and psychological functioning and therefore the ability to concentrate and relax. As long as a normal human being is willing, he or she may undergo hypnosis. Insusceptible people are simply not willing. There is a positive correlation between a person's willingness to relax and concentrate and the ability to undergo hypnosis.

Question: Do people under hypnosis go to sleep or become unconscious?

Answer: No. An individual should not expect to go to sleep. Hypnosis is a state of hyper-awareness that feels very relaxing. An individual is completely aware of everything that is occurring in the surrounding environment, as well as that which is happening in the inner mind. Hypnosis is a state of consciousness located somewhere between awake and asleep. Some fatigued people may go out of hypnosis by falling into natural sleep, simply because they are tired. In this case, if a person is trying to recall a memory, he or she can't do so while sleeping, so he or she needs to be awakened. On the other hand, if a person is listening to a self-hypnosis tape and falls out of hypnosis into sleep, the suggestions will likely still be effective. Sleep is also a learning state.

Question: What can be treated with hypnotherapy?

Answer: A qualified clinical hypnotherapist has the capabilities to help alleviate or transform a multitude of symptoms and problems. Many hypnotherapists carry credentials in other professional fields and therefore utilize hypnosis within the context of their specialty areas. For example, most clinical psychologists use hypnosis as an adjunct to psychotherapy methods. In contrast, a clinical hypnotherapist will use suggestive therapy, and sometimes regressive hypnosis, as the primary intervention to transform a problem or reach a therapeutic goal.

The more qualifying information clients seeking hypnotherapy services request (such as educational background, specialization, and the content of the treatment program) the better possibility they will choose a therapist who will appropriately match their needs and goals.

In summary, I believe that most of the misconceptions have been answered in this chapter. If there are other ones that surface, a good understanding of hypnosis on the part of the hypnotherapist can generally lead to helping potential clients become comfortable with the subject matter. Eliminating misconceptions increases rapport, which is a key factor to obtaining results. Resistance is often due to a client's misconceptions about hypnosis. Therefore, it is a good idea to help clients resolve these prior to, or at the beginning of, their first hypnotherapy session.

Chapter 7

Susceptibility to Hypnosis

Susceptibility refers to a person's ability to undergo hypnosis. Everybody is susceptible to hypnosis, because everybody enters into states of hypnosis a minimum of two times each day: when waking up from normal sleep; and when falling asleep. Waking hypnosis, or what is referred to as the hypnogogic state, is also inherent in human consciousness and occurs on a daily basis. Therefore, every person alive has a natural ability to enter into a state of hypnosis. If individuals were not able to undergo a state of hypnosis, then they must have an abnormal physiological or psychological condition that would serve to preventing them. Although everybody can undergo traditional forms of hypnosis, various right brain dominant populations, and certain personality types, are likely to be more susceptible to hypnosis.

Susceptible Populations

Children are the most susceptible to hypnosis. If we were to take into account the theory of personality formation presented by popular sociologist Morris Massey, we could theorize that a person's personality is not fully developed until the age of 21. According to Massey, the years between birth and age eight are the *imprint* years. Every "significant life event" (SLE) that occurs within these years becomes permanently imprinted upon the unconscious mind. There it stays as an impulse or unconscious behavior, unless it is accessed and transformed through a form of therapy, such as hypnosis, which accesses the unconscious mind.

Young children, during the imprint years, are in an altered state of consciousness the majority of the time. The subconscious is acutely open to suggestion, because the conscious or rational mind is not intercepting external information, in order to question it. In other words, young children experience their environment more directly, identifying with each situation presented.

Children are very imaginative, especially with story telling experiences. Children from about age three to ten can be told to close their eyes and imagine a story, in order to go into hypnosis. Milton Erickson understood the value of story telling for creating change with all of his clients. His understanding was that the mind works in a sequential fashion, so most thoughts create meaning in the mind by manifesting some form of a story.

Stories work particularly well with children, because of their natural ability for achieving identification. Identification is where an individual starts to identify with the characters of a story, even to the point of feeling the emotions and behaving the way the characters do after the story telling experience is over. People from age eleven and older tend to respond well to normal hypnotic inductions and suggestions.

People age fourteen to twenty-one are the most susceptible to hypnosis, according to Masud Ansari's book, *Modern Hypnosis.*[9] It appears that most of the people in this category go into hypnosis very quickly and easily. They also tend to experience hypnosis with a deeper trance level. As a result, the suggestions for change are very powerful. Although this particular age group is where a high number of problems in society originate, hypnotherapy is not yet a popular therapy for this population. Nonetheless, it is the most successful population for getting hypnotherapeutic results. For this reason, I predict that this therapeutic modality will eventually become the method of choice for this population in the future.

After the age of twenty-one, there is a steady decline in

susceptibility. However, this does not mean that the elderly make poor subjects. Success is primarily dependent on personality type and exposure. If an elderly person has an attitude of openness to new experiences, or has a productive belief in what hypnosis is and what it can do, he or she will generally undergo hypnosis easily. They simply have more mental associations (i.e. an idea reminds them of a story), and relative stories will often surface when considering the concept of hypnosis. In many cases, there is the need to patiently discuss more details that define hypnosis and the hypnotic experience, alleviating misconceptions.

Although it was believed at one time that women were more easily hypnotized, research shows that both sexes are equal in their ability to experience hypnosis. Research also indicates that certain personality types tend to be more susceptible, while others are less, as in the table below:

Table 7-1
Personality and Hypnotic Susceptibility

More	Less
Meditators	Engineers
Spiritualists	Scientists
Religious Types	Military Officers
Military Subordinates	Paranoids
Factory Workers	Investigators
Medicated Psychotics	Police Officials
Artists/Musicians	Extreme Analyticals

In general, those individuals that exercise a left brain dominance in their regular activities will tend to be less susceptible to hypnosis, while those who exercise right brain activities will tend to be more susceptible. All of those listed in the more susceptible list tend to have the ability to dissociate, or detach from their immediate environment and live within an imaginary inner-world.

Those in the less susceptible list tend to rationalize their world, predominantly using more of their left brain. Methods that may prove to be more successful would be those that are consistent with this population's normal way of using their imagination. For example, in order to induce hypnosis in a mechanical engineer, he or she could be told that his or her arms are on pulleys, and when the tension is let off of the pulley, the arms will relax. Although these things can help, there are also other ways that we can teach this population to pay attention to and experience their impressionistic-oriented subconscious mind. It is also important to keep in mind that not all of those listed in the less susceptible category are going to prove to be less susceptible. Many will prove to be good hypnosis clients, regardless of these generalizations.

Drugs and Hypnosis

Research shows that small amounts of narcotics and alcohol generally facilitate trance. In addition, I have found psychotropic drugs, antidepressants and the like, to also facilitate a state of hypnosis. The motivation level of those on psychotropics may need to be closely examined, however, when attempting hypnotherapeutic results.

Stimulants or amphetamines are counterproductive. One of the most common stimulants that seems to work against the process of hypnotic induction is caffeine. If a client has caffeine within a few hours before the session, he or she is likely to have difficulty entering into a state of hypnosis, and it may call for rescheduling the session for a day when the client can eliminate the use of caffeine beforehand.

Imaginability or "Suggestibility," (Syn.)

Imaginability simply refers to the extent to which a person can imagine an idea. It answers the question, "How much can I imagine this idea until I actually begin to experience it." There is a positive correlation between a subject's imaginability and: 1) his or her ability to efficiently undergo hypnosis, and 2) the depth of hypnosis achieved. People with a high imaginability factor are often right brain dominant, and because hypnosis is a right brain activity, a high imaginability factor indicates that an individual will be very successful with undergoing hypnosis.

Imaginability is a new term I've developed for the word "suggestibility," which has been historically used in hypnosis research to describe the same phenomenon. The reason I decided to update this terminology is because of the misconceptions associated with the old term. Suggestibility is perceived as gullibility by many. Instead, the word "imaginability," by nature, refers to a person's ability to imagine. Generally, the more imaginative an individual is, the more creative, intelligent, and successful, in the long run, within this ever-changing rapidly moving society. Certainly, as we will experience many times with clients of suggestive therapy, a person's ability to imagine desired outcomes increases the potential to achieve goals.

The following tests, listed and described below, generally measure just how imaginative a client may be, before attempting hypnosis. However, it is important to understand that imaginability tests can work both as: 1) convincers, proving that a person may effectively undergo a state of hypnosis; and 2) as stumbling blocks, proving that a person may not be able to undergo hypnosis. When clients fail an imaginability test, they may believe that they are insusceptible. For this reason, I recommend that these tests are only used for specific clients (which I will discuss later in this chapter) in a private practice setting. In groups, such as those in entertainment hypnosis, these tests are consistently used to choose subjects who will have more success performing the intended suggestions, selecting the most susceptible volunteers.

Imaginability Tests

1. Book and Balloon Test
2. Sway Test
3. Eye Catalepsy Test
4. Lemon Test
5. Car/House Memory Test
6. Pendulum Test

1) Book and Balloon Test- The hypnotherapist asks the client to hold out his or her hands, arms extended, with one palm facing up and the other facing down. He or she is instructed to close his or her eyes and imagine balloons being attached to the palm-down hand, and encyclopedias being placed on the palm-up hand. The balloon hand is being described by the therapist as getting lighter, with tugs and jerks from the balloons pulling upward, while the other hand is being described as getting heavier with each new encyclopedia that is placed upon it. Soon the distance between the hands increases, because the imagination is becoming more and more real to the body. This test is often used by entertainment hypnotists for determining the best subjects for the show; but it is also commonly used in private practice as well.

Book and Balloon Illustration

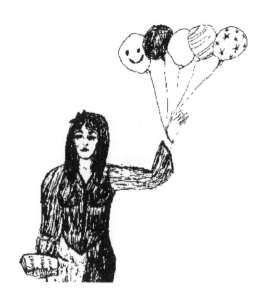

Note:
This individual has her eyes closed, imagining having a book resting on one hand and balloons tied to the other hand.

2) <u>Sway Test-</u> This is another test that is often used in enter-tainment hypnosis, both for its validity in imaginability and for its dramatic effect. The participants on stage are asked to close their eyes and imagine that they are swaying. They are instructed that when they are tapped on the shoulder, they should fall forward onto the hypnotist, who will catch them. Those who fall forward without stopping themselves pass the test. This primarily proves their trust level in that they will be caught by the hypnotist. This trust factor generally indicates a willingness to follow sugges-tions.

3) <u>Eye Catalepsy Test-</u> Subjects are told to close their eyes and imagine their "eyes are stuck closed." The subject is told to imagine that all of the muscles around the eyes are very relaxed and that a safe glue is put on the eyelids as they are closed. The glue is imagined as hardening during the hypnotist's counting to three. At the number three, the subject is told that the eye lids will be stuck together, and he or she can try to open them, but as hard as they try, they will remain stuck closed. The words, "stuck together" are repeated several times at the number three. Then, after only a few seconds, the individual is told that the glue is wiped off and the eyes may open naturally. The majority cannot seem to open their eyes, primarily because their thoughts are interrupted by the hypnotist's repetitive suggestion that the eye lids are stuck together.

4) <u>Lemon Test-</u> Subjects are told to imagine that they are in their kitchen safely cutting a wedge out of a big juicy lemon. Then, they imagine biting down into the lemon wedge as all of the juice squirts into the back of their mouths. Salivation is usually the re-sult, unless the client frequently eats lemons and is accustomed to the sour taste. About 90% of the public seems to salivate well with this test, which makes it one of my favorite. I always tell clients that with the power of their imagination, they have fooled their body into actually believing it needed to use a glandular function in order to digest the lemon. This is a good technique for those that are challenged with an illness, particularly if it involves the immune system. For example, a therapist could emphasize that

if a glandular function can be affected by imagery, then so can the immune system's ability to fight cancer. Dr. Carl Simonton, a prominent medical researcher, has shown the effectiveness of imagery to fight cancer in various studies and documented this in several books he has written on the subject.

5) Memory Regression Test- The memory test simply sets up parameters for a regression, when therapist and client are preparing for such an experience. It is an ideal procedure if the client has never experienced a hypnotic memory regression before. This test teaches the client what to expect, or what not to expect, if there is a misconception surrounding the memory regression experience. It can be performed with eyes open or closed as the client is told to think of his or her house or car.

Getting agreement that they are imagining such, subjects are then asked to describe "what angle" they see it from (front, back, etc.), and what they see, hear, and feel. This stimulates the three primary imagery channels of visual, auditory, and kinesthetic, and often indicates which one or two senses are dominant. The imagery becomes more clear and detailed, the longer the client describes it. Soon, he or she begins to relive the imagery as a memory. Often, it may be emphasized that there is something significant about the subject matter, such as a dent in the car or a favorite room in the house. This is a subconscious selection, and the importance of trusting the subconsciously selected imagery revolving around a specifically suggested subject matter is brought to the attention of the client. The hypnotherapist may encourage the client to "trust the subconscious" in the same way, while under hypnosis. This mind-set is likely to be the most important factor for achieving a hypnotic memory regression.

6) Pendulum Test- The subject is asked to hold a pendulum with the elbow supported on a table. The hypnotherapist asks the client's subconscious mind to indicate a "yes," "no," and perhaps a "maybe" answer. The pendulum will swing side-to-side or circle in a specific direction indicating a relational answer (e.g. a lateral swing indicates a "no" and a circular swing indicates a "yes'). This generally occurs through a person's fine motor muscles and the

unconscious mind. Because these movements are not detected by the conscious mind, the answer is generally deemed to be derived from the unconscious. This test is focused on asking a person's unconscious mind to give answers regarding his or her ability to undergo hypnosis, or the feasibility of a person's current therapeutic goal. In some applications, hypnotherapists use the pendulum for channeling spirit guidance, or accessing intuition, indicating that these directives are from the superconscious dimensions of mind.

The use of an imaginability test depends on personality type. It may be safely assumed that all subjects are good ones until proven otherwise. If a subject fails one or two tests, it may have a negative effect on induction. Nonetheless, some hypnotherapists rely on these tests regularly as an educational tool for themselves and their clients. As a result, they are generally more proficient at using them.

I believe that anyone can imagine what is suggested if only he or she is willing. The more relaxed and concentrated an individual is on the suggestions, the more likely he or she will be able to experience them and enter into hypnosis. I personally tend to use the tests as a teaching tool for a few select clients that appear in need of this form of hypnosis education, such as in the instances that follow.

Instances for Imaginability Tests

There are three conditions under which I will perform imaginability tests:

1) Previous unsuccessful experiences:

The client has had unsuccessful experiences with hypnosis. In this case, it is best to perform imaginability tests, in order to show the client that people must use their imagination to be able to experience hypnosis, and the resulting hypnotherapeutic successes. It is likely that these individuals had difficulties with using their imagination with another hypnotherapist, or imagery instructor, in the past.

2) <u>The prove-it-to-me personality type:</u>
The client doubts that he or she can be hypnotized and has a "prove it to me" type of attitude, which generally signifies a resistance. This resistance may exist because of a lack of understanding that imagination is the key to entering hypnosis, or they may be doubting and challenging the whole concept of being able to be hypnotized. The client may believe that he or she is insusceptible, or he or she may have underlying reasons to resist that are not apparent. This client-type typically reports that he or she is willing to change but cannot be hypnotized. Teaching these clients to use their imagination to obtain results, by using imaginability tests, may prove beneficial.

3) <u>The client lacks experience with regression:</u>
The hypnotherapeutic goal involves hypnotic regression, but the client has never experienced a regression before. In this case, the hypnotherapist can suggest the car / house memory regression test, which generally resolves misconceptions about regression. One of the most common misconceptions involves what I humorously refer to as the "beam me up Scotty" effect. This is where the client expects to be transported from one dimensional reality to another. Because of Hollywood movies, the client expects to regress and not know who they are in the present anymore. In actuality, hypnosis simply enhances a person's ability to recall information.

The ego, or conscious mind is still present during hypnotic regression and, in fact, serves as the action part of our consciousness. Without the conscious mind present in some way, it would be impossible for the client to verbalize the information surfacing in the subconscious mind to the hypnotherapist. The conscious mind is subdued, but must be present in order to make a hypnotic regression possible. For this reason, a medium to deep state of hypnosis is best for conducting a successful hypnotic memory regression, not somnabulism.

We will cover these and other concepts in later chapters designed to teach regression. For now, it is important to realize that clients need to be taught what to expect before performing hypnotic regression. This is often accomplished by discussing that which other clients have experienced in the past.

There are many reasons why clients do not pass imaginability tests. It is important to keep in mind that about 25% of individuals in the United States and Canada are not visually dominant, so their imagination process will involve more auditory and kinesthetic impressions. Others seem to try too hard, when the act of trying is a conscious mind activity, so they are destined to fail. Others may be afraid of hypnosis, don't have rapport with the hypnotherapist, or simply do not want the change that they claim they want. There are multiple reasons for resistance, and the chapter designated to such would be a good resource for further understandings.

Hypnosis can be metaphorically described as a big *magnifying glass*. Whatever an individual focuses on while under hypnosis becomes vivified, or lifelike. We can amplify the past for memory retrieval, or amplify the future for increasing motivation. In part, the subject begins to live the images because they are more vivid than the ones in the waking state. Because of this magnifying effect, clients who imagine the future the way they truly desire it will actually create a future memory, just as powerful as a past memory experience, and begin to live out their goal in that very moment. As a result, the motivation level dramatically increases. This is key to suggestive therapeutic success, because that which the mind can perceive, it can conceive.

Hypnotherapists must embrace the fact that we are *imagination therapists*. In other words, by utilizing a person's imagination, we are magnifying aspects of his or her mind and personality, and therefore able to implement change and transformation.

Chapter 8

Induction and Awakening Procedures

Four Eras of Hypnotic Induction

The <u>first era</u> of hypnosis (1784 to 1949) I refer to as the *experimental stage*. It spans from the time of Mesmer to the time of Freud. In these times, authoritarian styles were popular. Magnetism was thought by the masses to be Mesmerism, or a form of hypnotic suggestion. Clients that did not respond to basic techniques were thought to be insusceptible, as was claimed by Freud during his experimentation. The practitioner's tools and techniques were very limited and so were their capabilities.

The <u>second era</u> of hypnosis (1950-1979) I refer to as the *mixed era*. It includes the popular stage shows in the 1950s, the hypnotic childbirth era in the 1960s, and a marginal loss of popularity in the 1970s. Eye fixation and other physical induction methods, such as tapping on the forehead, looking into the eyes, and staring at a swinging watch, were prevalent for inducing hypnosis. Therefore, rapid induction was the method of choice. Although eye fixation methods were effective, they also carried connotations of being magical, or entertainment oriented, in the public eye. A mixture of methods for obtaining concentration, such as pendulums, swinging watches, spiraling disks, hour glasses, and even staring at a light bulb, or spots on the wall, were used to gain the attention of the subject. It was also thought by the vast majority of hypnotists and hypnotherapists that the tiring of the eyes was necessary for producing a hypnotic state. However, this began changing in the latter part of this time span with the introduction of Milton Erickson's methodology, which started bringing hypnotherapy back into the mainstream of society as being a viable therapeutic modality.

In the third era of hypnosis (1980-1999), which I refer to as the *education era*, hypnotherapists began to recognize that hypnosis was an altered state of consciousness that individuals automatically entered by daydreaming, driving on the highway, reading a book, listening to an interesting story, or watching an interesting television program. Erickson referred to this as waking hypnosis. Hypnotherapists began to recognize that tiring of the eyes was effective, yet unnecessary, for achieving a state of hypnosis. It became understood that a sequence of images produced hypnosis. Eye tiring practices to gain concentration are bypassed by simply asking the subject to close his or her eyes. From there, images are suggested so that the subject can relax and enjoy them. As a result, the attention span is substantially lengthened.

In the fourth era of hypnosis (2000 to 2100), which is referred to as the *Aquarian Era*, the *future* of hypnosis may be described as a daily occurrence that is recognized as the natural and simple fact that we, as human beings, undergo self-hypnotic states of mind that can be utilized to our advantage on a daily basis. As a result of this almost universal acceptance, I predict that forms of hypnosis will be taught to the general public, and as most individuals become aware of the daily and practical benefits, it will be utilized by the majority of individuals.

By the year 2050, I expect that most people will understand the natural triggers that allow them to undergo various levels of the altered state. These will be productively utilized for a wide variety of common purposes. Chemoanesthesia will become as uncommon as hypnoanesthesia is today. Accelerated learning will be taught to school children through trance states, and learning will become more enjoyable to children. The educational system will incorporate all learning styles through the in-depth understanding of the subconscious and unconscious minds.

Stress will be alleviated through a daily regime of self-hypnosis within those establishments currently referred to as corporate and government. The concept of "memory" will change dramatically and will begin to lose its current importance for self identity and instead portray a sense of in-the-now awareness. Past traumas will be alleviated with hypnotherapy as the obvious method of choice. Hypnosis will also be preferred for specific physiological changes, or healing, when combined with intention. Biochemical shifts, such as those experienced in the immune system, the circulatory system, and various cells and tissues in the body, will be seen as being more easily affected through scientifically researched forms of hypnosis. Specific cycles per second brain wave activity— primarily beta, alpha, theta, and delta—will become correlated with mental, spiritual, and physical healing; then eventually these brain waves will become scientifically exacted and utilized to produce more predictable outcomes relative to our connection to nature, individual healing, and other spiritual dimensions.

By the turn of the 22nd century (2100), the human culture on earth will become completely aware of the productive uses of various subtle levels of altered states of consciousness. These will be fully ingrained in society as the norm for many valuable functions. An ignorance of the uses of hypnosis will seem awkward and unusual. Finding the well-known, acceptable and productive trance levels within the self will be a natural process of education facilitated from birth onwards for each human being, regardless of cultural background. Mechanical shortcuts will be used for specific treatment methods for achieving effective psychological, physiological, and spiritual states of mind. With expanded awareness and the commonality of daily altered states, most will be able to reach these levels with quick, readily available, self-hypnosis methodologies.

Preparation For Induction

There are three primary factors that involve posture which need to be addressed by every hypnotherapist and client. These factors should be taught to the client either in the interview process as the last subject discussed before induction, or as the first few sentences at the beginning of an induction, (e.g. "Close you eyes now and get your back into a comfortable position that it can stay in for a period of time. Then, separate you hands to reduce distractions, and uncross your legs to reduce discomfort that could arise in the hip, knees, or ankles.").

Once these factors are addressed, hypnotic induction and a continuous adequate trance-level throughout the session is better insured.

Back- The back needs to be in a straight position. The hypnotherapist should help the client reduce slouching by avoiding curved-back chairs. It is wise to have a well padded chair as well. The middle of the back may need to be supported, if the chair is curved. The best chair to use is a recliner, because it is client centered. The client can recline as far back as he or she feels is comfortable.

Hands- The hands need to be separated to reduce the common distraction of touching the hands or fingers together and twiddling. This activity takes the concentration away from the hypnotherapist's words, and then the client begins to create his or her own subject matter to focus upon, such as a current daily stress.

Legs- The legs need to be uncrossed at the knees and ankles. Crossing the legs may initially make the client feel comfortable for the first few minutes, but after several minutes pain will enter into the joints from strain. When this occurs, the client will either remain uncomfortable, not saying anything, or have to uncross them to get more comfortable, potentially causing a disturbance in the trance.

Correct Body Posture

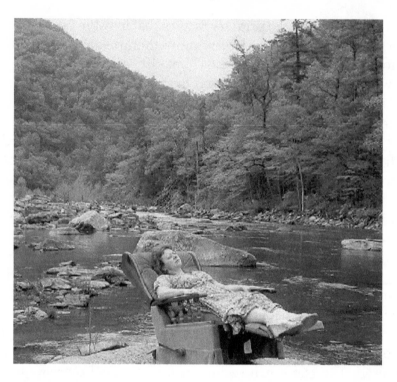

Note: The person in the illustration was instructed to separate her hands and feet, put her back into a straight position, and close her eyes to imagine she is relaxing in a "safe place"—a mountainous river bed.

Preparing the Environment

Although the back, legs, and hands, are the most important factors for a client and hypnotherapist to consider before attempting hypnotic induction, there are many other important factors that may arise. Although a few of these involve unique conditions of the client's body, most of these factors involve the office environment. When a client is comfortable, and the environment is adjusted properly, the chances for a successful induction are increased.

Eyes- It is best if eye wear is removed, since glasses and contacts can have an irritable effect on the eyes or nose, which gets amplified with hypnosis and causes a disturbance in the trance.

Bodily Functions- An individual using the bathroom before he or she undergoes hypnosis may be a good idea, since this particular need, if present, may also get amplified during trance when focused upon. In addition, tearing or crying may also occur. It is wise to keep a box of tissues next to the client, so that the client may utilize it when necessary. In these cases, it is best that a hypnotherapist give the client a tissue, warning the client of this form of touching beforehand, so that a startle is not encountered.

Temperature- Because the body temperature drops during hypnosis, there is a necessity to keep the temperature at or around 75 degrees. As a general rule, if the hypnotherapist feels a little warm, the temperature is probably adequate for the client. Body temperature drops with trance, as it does during natural sleep at bedtime, and it generally raises with the use of covers.

Scents- Often smells have associations. It is a good idea to check with the client to find out what scents, if any, he or she believes to be relaxing. This aspect of client centered hypnotherapy is important, as it also is for effective aromatherapy.

Sounds- Similar to the above, it's best to check with the client to find out what background music or sounds the client subjectively finds to be pleasing. Remaining client centered in the selection process can avoid various forms of resistance.

Lighting- Dim lighting is ideal for facilitating the production of imagery. If the lights are too bright, then a bright red effect in the mind's eye detracts. This is because of the blood in the eyelids. If it is completely dark, then the mind's eye may be too black to produce imagery. It may be best to either use easily adjustable window shades, or a dimmer switch, to create the moderate dim lighting that is optimal for achieving success.

Moods- Moods can often detract if they are unrelated to the hypnotherapy goal. However, if the mood stems from the goal, it will produce a deeper trance level, as individuals tend to be entranced with their problems.

If the mood is due to a subject matter that is unrelated to the therapeutic goal, it is hard for the client to concentrate on that which is being suggested during the induction. If the mood is related to the therapeutic topic, then it facilitates the hypnotherapy session.

Unrelated negative moods and topics are difficult to ignore and are best confronted and resolved before moving forward with a hypnosis session.

Handicaps- If an individual is hard of hearing, it will be beneficial for the hypnotherapist to speak louder during the interview and sit closer to the subject during the induction. The natural tendency of the therapist to speak softly will need to be consciously avoided throughout the session. Other considerations for handicapped individuals may include selecting an office on the ground floor to avoid steps, and having a rest room qualified for the handicapped.

Four Factors of Induction

Induction is the process whereby individuals enter into hypnosis. Hypnotic induction involves four primary factors that create an altered state of consciousness. These factors are used, in some way, by the majority of hypnotherapists for every induction. When they are present, the success rate of an induction is higher.

1) Concentration
2) Relaxation
3) Suggestion
4) Expectation

1) Concentration is the only factor that is a prerequisite for producing a successful hypnotic induction. If all of the other factors are present, and concentration is not, producing hypnosis is impossible. Once concentration is obtained, the doorways to suggestion are sustained for as long as the concentration level is maintained.

To further experience levels of concentration, consider the following concentration exercises:

a) Closed Eye Fixation- To try this exercise, readers may simply close their eyes and blank their mind until they get a thought. At the onset of any thought at all, they should refocus their mind on blanking again for as long as possible. Readers should see how long they can keep the mind blank. It will usually last only seconds. Some well practiced meditators can blank their mind longer than others.

b) Opened Eye Fixation- Readers should stare at a spot somewhere in the room and blank their mind. At the onset of any thought at all, readers should refocus on blanking their mind for as long as possible. Readers should see how long they can blank their mind. It is generally easier to blank the mind using the environment.

c) Moving Object- Readers may use an hour glass, a swinging watch, or some moving object to stare at, and eventually they will find themselves staring through the object, relaxing and blanking their mind. At the onset of any thought at all, it is important to refocus on blanking the mind for as long as possible. Readers should see how long they can blank their mind. It is generally easier to blank the mind for longer periods of time using moving objects.

d) Imagery- Readers may close their eyes and imagine a favorite vacation or a any desirable place. It may be a real place or simply an imagined one. Most people prefer to focus on nature. Readers should try to stay focused on all of the details in the mind's eye. When they have filled in the sights, sounds, and senses, they will notice how much longer they have been able to concentrate on the scene as it progresses. Readers may find the movement in the scene to be most interesting and captivating.

Most people will find imagery as the most effective tool for lengthening their concentration levels. The next most effective tool is a moving object. Thereafter, opened eye and closed eye fixation tend to be equally less effective on the average, but practice makes perfect. In addition, it is important to keep in mind that eye fixation methods used to lengthen concentration and induce hypnosis tend to be associated with entertainment hypnosis or old-school hypnosis. Most modern schools of hypnotherapy teach imagery as part of the hypnotic induction.

2) <u>Relaxation</u> generally deepens a person's trance level. With deeper relaxation, the subject's imagination is more vivid and

more compelling. Suggestions to relax the whole body are generally effective for inducing hypnosis. When the body is relaxed, the conscious mind's critical sensor slows, or becomes pacified, so that the subconscious mind, the part of the mind that uses images to communicate, can become more active. The sound of the hypnotherapist's voice is also an important factor for helping a client relax with suggestions.

3) <u>Suggestion</u> is necessary to direct the state of relaxed concentration toward a specific goal. In reference to induction, suggestion is primarily made up of words that describe relaxing concepts or images. In reference to therapy, suggestions create images that are relevant to the therapeutic goal. Selecting words that are associated with relaxation is most important for induction.

4) <u>Expectation</u> is important on both sides of the hypnotherapeutic relationship. Understanding our client's expectations and attempting to fulfill them increases the chance that therapeutic goals will become realized. If the subject is expecting to go to sleep, he or she often will do so during the session. In this case, if the person does indeed fall asleep, it often fulfills his or her expectations.

I remember a client who worked with a psychologist in the western United States before she moved east to do hypnotherapy with me. When I was in the middle of my induction, she opened her eyes and claimed that she was not being hypnotized. I then asked how she was successfully hypnotized in the past, and she said that her former hypnotherapist used eye fixation. I positively agreed that fixation was a valid method, secretly knowing that it was outdated, and then I proceeded to copy the method through her description. As she stared at a spot on the wall for approximately five minutes, I was still. Her eyes became tired and red and then she closed them. Immediately, I began to apply suggestions of relaxation and deepening, and her hypnotherapeutic goal for a regression was a success.

It is important for a hypnotherapist to exercise patience when working to induce hypnosis in a client. Patience, as we've just read about above, increases success. Just as important for achieving induction is the hypnotherapist's side of the "faith factor," or the expectation of the hypnotherapist. A client will only go into themselves in the places that we imagine are possible.

In order to induce hypnosis, bypassing the critical factor is necessary. The critical factor is known as the conscious mind. This is the part of the mind that rationalizes, analyzes, and makes decisions about the internal and external environment. Another term used in better describing the effect is *pacification*; to pacify the conscious mind with suggestions that are simple and relaxing.

Once pacified, the conscious mind becomes subdued, or less active, and the subconscious mind becomes predominant. During a successful hypnotic induction, suggestions begin to go directly into the subconscious and unconscious areas of mind, with less interception from the conscious mind.

Mind Circles Illustration

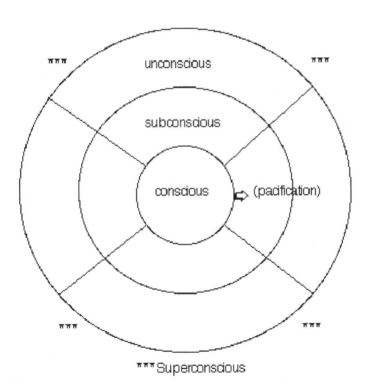

Methods of Hypnotic Induction

What follows are three primary categories of hypnotic induction. All inductions fall under these three methods.

Physical induction methods utilize physical forms of relaxation involving objective, observable forms of relaxation. Some techniques that fall under this category include suggestions such as, "Feel all of the facial muscles relax now, as the jaw un-clenches." This can be studied objectively as a hypnotherapist watches the muscle tone in the face change.

A popular physical induction method is known as progressive relaxation. In this method, the hypnotherapist tells the client to relax from the top of the head to the tip of the toes, or visa versa. The client focuses on each part of the body as he or she imagines it relaxing, until the whole body becomes relaxed. This method is ideal for teaching self-hypnosis to those with sleeping problems. Once the clients lay down to sleep, they may perform a progressive relaxation on themselves and thereby fall asleep rather quickly.

Psychic induction methods are more subjective, because they involve mental or psychological forms of relaxation that are unique to that individual. For example, one person may consider the beach to be relaxing, while another may not because of a near drowning experience. A background tape may be used with nature sounds on it as part of an induction. These are all subjective approaches, so if a hypnotherapist decides to use background sounds, it may be best to pre-qualify these methods with a client before attempting them.

The best psychic methods include describing common nature imagery that is generally found to be relaxing for the majority of the general public. This can save both hypnotherapist and client the effort of pre-qualifying.

Psychophysical induction methods include a mix of psychic and physical relaxation techniques. The *mixed method* is the most widely used induction method today. Generally, this method involves progressive relaxation and popular forms of imagery (oceans, mountains, etc.). Combining these two methods into one increases the probability of achieving success with a broader range of personality types.

The best inductions include expanded psychic methods, utilizing the five sensory modalities of see, hear, feel, taste and smell (visual, auditory, kinesthetic, gustatory, and olfactory). These generally facilitate imagery to be more compelling. Since people tend to be dominant in two or three of these modalities, they will experience those senses as a hypnotherapist describes them and ignore the others. Describing the most common three (seeing, hearing, and feeling) tend to be adequate for success. In the process, a progressive relaxation may be worked into the induction to insure the broad spectrum effect that most personality types require for success.

I have several inductions that I use for various reasons, yet the one I rely upon the most with the majority of my clients, due to its broad spectrum capability, is the Safe Place Induction. It offers a level of psychic effectiveness that is not generally found in other inductions, as it suggests that individuals find a place where they feel safe in nature. It has been taken from two historical clinical uses: the hospitalized patient who has been bed ridden for a long period of time; and the recovering abused child.

In the case where a patient has been bed ridden for a long period of time, and he or she is experiencing stress and anxiety, the patient can imagine that he or she is somewhere else. This beneficial level of dissociation has proven to be very therapeutic. In cases of children with post traumatic stress from abuse, and they have no reference for feeling safe, these children have been able to successfully develop a safe place in their mind from being taught safe place imagery. Once the children had subjectively learned to feel safe again, mental health professionals have utilized these imaginary places as a foundation for recovery.

In my sharing an induction with readers, I am assuming that they will not utilize the induction on others without proper formal training in clinical hypnosis (see the Afterword to find resources for such). The lack of formal training would not only result in inefficiency, but it may also result in complications for the client. In the following Safe Place Induction, notice that the imagery segment, the first paragraph, contains the psychic portion of the mixed method, and the progressive relaxation portion, (the next two paragraphs), involves the physical. It is in the psychic portion where four out of five sensory modalities are found, in effort to further broaden the induction and satisfy most personality types. Also notice that the induction may be utilized with a broad range of deepening techniques—which may be derived from the chapter on deepening and may be inserted at the segment indicating "deepening techniques..." near the end of the induction. In addition, the area outlining, "therapy..." after deepening techniques is the point where therapy scripts may be inserted which are related to the client's goal:

Safe Place Induction

Safe Place Imagery...

Separate your hands and feet and put your back into a comfortable position that it can stay in for a long period of time. Close your eyes and allow yourself to imagine a safe place in nature where you've been before or plan to be, or you may just create it within yourself. Brighten up the color and notice how clear it is and how good it feels to be there. Notice the things that are moving about and how peaceful and wonderful the mood is. Hear the sounds of nature now, as they get a little louder. You may feel the warmth of the light in the sky, and the coolness of a gentle breeze. There may be a familiar scent in the air...a few clouds drifting gently across the sky, a sky that goes on forever and a bright light that reaches you shining down between the clouds allowing you to feel warm and relaxed. This light stands for everything that's good in life, such as love, peace, serenity, tranquility, and pure relaxation.

Progressive Relaxation...

Allow this light to flow through relaxing every muscle fiber, cell and tissue. As it flows through you from head to toe, allow it to completely relax each muscle group. As it begins to flow through the forehead, feel the stress lines simply spread apart. It automatically continues to flow through the eyes as the thread muscles behind the eyes simply unravel and the eyes get heavier. The white light automatically continues to flow down over the temples and through the front of the neck...at the same time down the back of the head, neck and shoulders. Allow gravity to pull the shoulders down into their natural position. The mind may wander and drift, or it may become drowsy and foggy. Whatever happens is completely natural; you'll still hear the relaxing sound of my voice which is soon to become a comfortable feeling in the background. My words will soon blend into one another and flow into your mind naturally, so you'll be free from having to listen to the words as the subconscious will recognize what they mean anyway. And the mind simply unwinds like a big spring...letting go. As the sun rises on one side of the earth and sets on the other, each day is similar to one another with common themes. Each day has learning lessons of its own, regardless of the ups and down, moods, stresses...it has nothing to do with this. This is just pure-simple relaxation. All fears, guilts and self blame are released. Problems, pressures, and stresses built up through time are useless and unnecessary.

Allow the white light to continue to flow through the elbows, wrists, and out through the fingers. You may notice a tingling sensation within the hands which further shows you're beginning to relax as the bodily functions are slowing down. The breathing becomes a shade deeper; with each more relaxing breath, feel the body rest more firmly against the pads that you're laying or sitting against. As the white light flows down through the back, all the muscles and tendons wrapped around the vertebrae unwind, and the back settles into its natural position automatically. The light flows through the waist, knees, ankles, and out through the toes, pushing out all stress, concerns, worries, in the form of tension or tightness, which may have been locked up in the body and are useless to us now. Feel the nerves dimming, like dimming the lights. And with each beat of the heart, that you're naturally more in touch with from becoming relaxed in this way, allow yourself to go deeper into relaxation. Feel all the muscles and tendons droop and hang on the bone structure, loose and limp.

Deepening techniques...

Therapy...

Awakening Procedures...
And now I'm going to count back from five to one and when I reach the number one, you can then normalize.

> *Five*...You'll remember everything you have experienced.
> *Four*...Very satisfied (with changes that have taken place).
> *Three*...More in touch with the room around you.
> *Two*...The mind and the body are returning back toward normal.
> When you imagine the number *One* in your mind's eye within the next minute, you'll become wide awake, refreshed; and feeling good.

Induction scripts- These scripts are the most valuable tool for a hypnotherapist, particularly for the beginning hypnotherapist. The reading of scripts is hidden from clients, since they generally have their eyes closed. After a period of time, the experienced hypnotherapist will have memorized their induction script(s) from regular use and abandon them (not suggestive therapy scripts, as these are difficult to memorize). The best induction scripts are designed for a variety of personality types. If the student of hypnotherapy does not have scripts to use along with this book, it may be best to obtain another book that I wrote titled, *Script Magic: A Hypnotherapist's Desk Reference*, which contains over one hundred scripts that include hypnotic induction, deepening, suggestive therapy, and methods of regression .

Time Factor- A new client's first induction should be a *formal induction*. This type of induction should take about 15 to 20 minutes. The primary benefit of formal induction involves clients learning a variety of relaxation concepts that will generally reduce stress in their every day lives and on a regular basis. This occurs from clients repetitively listening to the induction and subsequently remembering the relaxation exercises within it.

In addition, most researchers agree that the longer the induction time, the more likely it is that the client will be hypnotized, and the deeper will be the state of hypnosis achieved. Therefore, for these reasons, I recommend the formal induction over quicker methods, such as rapid induction.

Once a client has experienced a few hypnotherapy sessions, the hypnotherapist may choose to shorten the induction time. Rapid or instantaneous inductions, or some other advanced induction methods, which are outlined in next chapter, may be used, because of the increased conditioning of the client. One advantage to this is that hypnotherapist and client may save time. Once clients are conditioned to the hypnotherapist's voice and office surroundings, a shorter induction tends to be just as effective as the formal induction. A shortened version of the formal induction may also serve to be adequate.

Awakening Procedures

I recommend against quick methods, such as snapping fingers, clapping aloud, etc., because it may be unpleasant and startle the client, particularly when he or she is in a deep trance. Instead, it is best to bring the client back slowly and peacefully, including suggestions of well being. The deeper the trance level, the slower that the awakening procedures should be performed.

In general, it is best to bring the client back from trance by counting back from 5 to 1, because of the rocket or shuttle association that we have from watching the space program on television, i.e.. "five, four, three, two, one, blast off!." I also prefer to build into the awakening procedures one final post hypnotic suggestions at "four," for the purpose of increasing therapeutic success. The following are the *awakening procedures* that I tend to use regularly:

Five... You'll remember everything.

Four... Wonderfully satisfied as a _____(e.g. nonsmoker).

Three... More in touch with the room around you now.

Two... The mind and body are returning back to normal with all of the natural changes that have taken place.

...and when you imagine the number one in your mind's eye within the next minute or less, you will become wide awake and refreshed with a beautiful sense of well being.

If the clients are not dehypnotized upon the use of the awakening procedures, there generally is no danger. They will eventually either awaken by themselves in a short period of time or drop off into natural sleep, dependent on their normal sleep schedule. However, in some cases, the client is purposely avoiding the suggestions to awaken. What follows are possible causes for this resistance:

Causes of Resistance to Dehypnotization
1. A desire to rebel against the hypnotherapist
2. A desire to deny the hypnotherapist's suggestions to awaken
3. The subject is not willing to carry out a post hypnotic suggestion
4. The subject is not willing to give up a pleasant feeling
5. The subject is avoiding a difficult life stress
6. The subject spontaneously lapsed back into hypnosis
7. The subject's fatigue causes them to sleep

Awakening resistance occurs infrequently. However, if a subject resists awakening, there are three main procedures that may be implemented to produce awakening:

1) Raise your voice and say, "____, you can wake up now!"

2) Say, "____, if you don't awaken now, you will take up more time and it will be more costly for you."

3) Avoid touching the client if at all possible; however, as a last resort, a hypnotherapist may raise and drop the hand, and as the hand hits the furniture say, "Wake up!"

Touching- Although early forms of hypnotic inductions involved touching, this is not recommended today, unless the practitioner has other credentials that would indicate that touching is customary (e.g. massage therapist, healing touch or reiki practitioner, etc.). Touching as a hypnotherapy practitioner may cause a startle, for several reasons: because of a person's being in a deeply relaxed state of mind; because of a lack of rapport; because of a client's past experiences with inappropriate contact; and more.

I have learned to touch only with permission prior to contact, or at the client's request. However, as I've mentioned earlier, in the cases where the client has tears streaming down his or her face, I will inform the client that I am going to put a tissue in his or her hand. At this, only about half of the clients use the tissue.

Post session interview

At the end of the session, I will often leave the client alone for a few minutes so that they can gather their normal faculties. I may leave the room and get a drink, or simply turn away in silence and write a few simple notes about the session and a receipt for payment, indicating the amount of their bill. I save this for the very last topic. Then, I ask the client how they are doing.

Sometimes upon awakening, clients just want to pay and leave. Sometimes clients have a few comments on how they felt about doing hypnosis. Sometimes, particularly if they have just experienced a hypnotic regression, there will be a need to talk about what the client encountered. Most clients, however, only need about 5 minutes to talk, and then they are happy to leave. Sometimes, if a client seems to want to talk longer than I have time for, due to my next scheduled appointment, and it is simply chitchat, or it can wait until the next session, I will stand up and start talking about something unrelated to the session, the weather, or what the client is going to do later in the day. These steps graduate a person into normal thinking and help to speed up the process of mentally shifting gears. With some individuals that are still "spacey," it may be best to ask the client to sit down in the waiting room, until he or she feels comfortable leaving or driving.

Sometimes I ask the client if he or she would like a hug, particularly if the client had an emotional experience, and if there is good rapport. However, there should never be any need on the part of the hypnotherapist for this; and it should only be done with the client's need in mind. This ensures that a clinical relationship is perceived and maintained. A hug is best when initiated by the client. Two other appropriate methods of affection include cradling their hand with both of yours and shaking lightly, or reaching out and shaking with one hand while placing the other hand on the back of their shoulder.

If a client is in a program with a predetermined number of sessions, then it's as some native Americans have been known to say when parting, "Until we meet again," at their next scheduled appointment. If the client is not scheduled for another appointment, then I generally leave it up to him or her to call my office to make another date to see me. This is part of the client centered approach.

In summary, formal induction, under the mixed method, is generally the most effective for the majority of hypnotherapy clients; therefore it is the most commonly used induction. Yet, when students of hypnotherapy become more experienced, they may find that, under certain conditions, other inductions have superior benefits. For the purpose of gaining a better education in hypnotherapy, these will be discussed in the next chapter.

Chapter 9

Advanced Induction Methods

When considering how to create and utilize an effective hypnotic induction , a hypnotherapist needs to include enhancement tools. The tools listed below will enhance any particular induction method:

1) Trance Voice
2) Pacing
3) Semantics
4) Deepening Techniques
5) Protective Suggestions

Trance Voice- This is probably the best way to enhance an induction script. The trance voice is very different from a normal speaking voice. In trance voice, the speaker softens his or her words, like a mother speaking to a child at bedtime. A trance voice also includes speaking from the diaphragm. An example of the best breathing technique would be how a singer sings from his or her diaphragm, reducing the amount of air that passes through the nasal passages. Some singers claim the effect to be like a balloon full of air and pinching the opening so that the air escapes at a constant rate. Taking a deep breath and slowly but steadily exhaling the words while half talking and half whispering is the key to obtaining the trance voice.

Pacing- This effect is accomplished by reading off a certain number of words from an induction script with each exhale. There is a pause on the inhale, and then another series of words is spoken again on the exhale. These words may end in the middle of a sentence or at the end of a sentence, depending on where the hypnotherapist ends his or her breath. The key is to use the same relaxed pace of breathing with each exhale and expel approximately the same number of words or syllables. This steady pace of breathing and speaking has been shown to slow the pace of thoughts and breaths of the client, as he or she unconsciously paces the hypnotherapist's rhythms.

Semantics- All suggestions should involve words that are positive and simple, in order to increase success. Positive semantics are a general rule of thumb for designing induction scripts, as well as designing suggestions for therapy. If the words are simple enough for a young child to understand, then they will likely be suitable for the subconscious mind as well. Semantics that are outcome-based are also best, describing clients' positive goals, rather than the stresses that we don't want them to experience in the future. Positive and simple semantics are contained in the best induction scripts.

Deepening Techniques- These techniques, which will be further studied in a subsequent chapter, are very effective when they are built into induction scripts. One such deepening technique that could essentially be included in every induction script is deep breathing exercises. These exercises consist of relaxing the body more deeply with each breath, (e.g. "With each breath you will go deeper"). Rapid induction requires deepening techniques to be effective. Deepening techniques are always best as part of any induction.

Protective Suggestions- This type of suggestion is used to protect a state of hypnosis from being disrupted. Because hypnosis is a natural amplifier, anything may be amplified during a state of hypnosis, including a client's external environment. If there is a loud sound, and the client chooses to perceive it as "disturbing," then it will be magnified as a significant disturbance. Likewise, it can be perceived as nothing, or better yet, as a signal to relax even further. My favorite protective suggestion that I use with almost every client is, "All outside sounds are signals for you to relax more deeply." This suggestion can be used in two places during a session: at the beginning of the induction script; or at any time during the induction, as the hypnotherapist deems necessary. Generally, protective suggestions are very effective, unless loud disturbing sounds remain persistent (e.g. a buzz saw used for remodeling the office while a hypnotherapy session is in progress). At that point, the source of the noise must be eliminated. In those rare instances, the hypnotic induction can be started over, if necessary.

Advanced Induction Methods

It is important to recognize that the induction methods listed below are not superior to a formal induction, in the vast majority of cases. An advanced induction method is recommended to be utilized only under specific circumstances. They are as follows:

1) Disguised Induction
2) Story Telling Induction
3) Rapid Induction
4) Affect Bridge Induction

The Disguised Induction was first introduced by Milton Erickson. According to Erickson, hypnosis cannot be resisted if no (apparent) hypnosis is detected. This method was developed because the word *hypnosis* has certain stigmas, which may prevent skeptical individuals from trying it. Because of this, an individual may not reap the benefits of this naturally occurring altered state, unless the practitioner refers to it as something else. Because hypnosis is a common daily experience, it can be given several other labels, such as an "imagery exercise," a "relaxation exercise," a "story," an "imagination game," and so on. Because hypnosis truly is all of these things and more, the practitioner can encourage others to try the experience.

The traditional disguised method is generally not recommended for one primary reason—truthfulness brings about a greater power, and power in the right hands manifests transformation. Truthfulness is a virtue that becomes instilled automatically within others by its use. People are living within an intuitive age right now, so they can perceive if others are truthful or not. Also, this virtue within a therapist automatically encourages clients to become truthful with themselves and their adversities.

The only time that this method is recommended is when someone is so anxious about hypnosis that they need to be taught its components in segments before trying the complete induction. For example, for those that have problems feeling out of control, with anxiety or panic attacks, hypnosis can be perceived as a threat as well as a benefit. Often the thought of being under hypnosis brings about panic, and a resulting cancellation or an appointment no-show. Yet, these clients wish very much to muster up the courage to try hypnosis and reap its transformative benefits. As a result, I tell these individuals that there will be no hypnosis used on the first session, just a consultation regarding their stresses and anxieties. However, at the end of the first session, relaxation techniques I refer to as "safe place imagery" and "progressive relaxation" are offered, and the client generally accepts. This could be referred to as a form of hypnosis, because it has components of a hypnotic induction and produces a light altered state. Yet, it *is* different, in that it is not as deep, since there are no deepening techniques used. This ambiguity makes it a form of the disguised method.

Story Telling Inductions, or metaphors, are Ericksonian in origin. Erickson used stories as metaphors for a variety of therapeutic goals. These stories often were used to have the client identify with the characters in the story, resulting in dissociation and a trance state. At some point, the story would change so that the characters experienced a resolution of the problem that would be symbolic of the therapeutic goal.

Sometimes stories can be used specifically to induce a trance. With a trance voice and a relaxing story, almost anybody can become relaxed, and in many cases very deeply. Stories can also be used as parts of other inductions, such as somebody walking on the beach and having a very relaxing experience. Telling short stories of success may be used during the client interview to elicit certain states within clients, like confidence, which may be useful for reaching therapeutic goals. This may be accomplished by telling the client about another client, name unmentioned, who had a similar problematic condition and was successful at changing it. These stories have the full power of indirect suggestion.

Rapid Induction, is also referred to in some texts as instantaneous induction. It is an induction that occurs very rapidly, compared to a formal induction. It will generally start with eye fixation, in order to gain concentration, and is followed by eye closure. Then, it is followed up with several deepening techniques in succession. Generally, it will take only one to five minutes to put a volunteer under hypnosis.

Rapid induction is often used in a group. Many stage hypnotists use this method, because it is quick, looks dramatic, and is effective with more susceptible personalities. However, because there is very little clinical value, in comparison to a formal induction which contains stress release and relaxation methods, it is generally not used in private practice settings. It may, however, be used by those who have a heavy client load and very little time for each client, such as a physician. It may also be used effectively by emergency medical personnel, because the conscious mind of an injured person is scrambled during emergencies, which makes them very susceptible to hypnosis and open to suggestion. In addition, many hypnotherapy trainers use it to save time during course instruction.

Affect Bridge Induction, or what some texts refer to as "somatic bridge," is a concept that originated from the work of Fritz Perls. He discovered that significant ideas and emotions expressed through normal conversation were often at the end of a gestalt. A gestalt is a series of events locked in the unconscious as memories, which culminate in a symptom or problem of the current day. These symptoms are represented with certain semantics or emotions, which are expressed and tagged by the hypnotherapist during a client interview. Once the beginning of the gestalt is found, by regressing the client back to the first memory which caused the problem, the rest of the trigger events which occurred thereafter (all the way up through the present) are resolved.

Emotional bridges are the easiest way to find the beginning of a gestalt. Because emotions are part of the unconscious mind, they can serve as a window to instantly bridge the subject into a causative root memory. These bridges may be discovered through the words or feelings that a client describes mentally or physically. At that point, the client is asked to close his or her eyes and "go back to the cause" or "remember the first time you began feeling this way", or "go back to the source of this problem."

This method is advised against, unless the student of hypnotherapy has been trained in advanced levels of hypnotic regression therapy. Thereafter, this method should only be utilized if clients have undergone regression before and they are, therefore, well familiarized with the process of regression; otherwise, it may not produce the desired effect, particularly when there exists short term and inadequate levels of rapport. For this reason, I always use a formal induction for a first-time hypnotic regression client. At some point in time, however, if a client has had several successful regressions, affect bridge can save time and be very effective.

To summarize...as a general rule, it is advisable to use formal induction, as opposed to advanced inductions, with the vast majority of clients. This is due to the fact that a formal induction, as indicated in the previous chapter, gives clients therapeutic benefits that are unique to the mixed method. In other words, using psychic and physical forms of relaxation teaches clients how to relax. This training not only occurs in the "trance chair" (the recliner that clients use in the office) but also at home and in their everyday lives. When clients want to use self-hypnosis to relax on work breaks or at home, the stress relief benefits are still available to them, as they remember the imagery or the relaxation exercises that they experienced in the hypnotherapy office. In addition, clients often listen to the formal induction at home on a self-hypnosis tape; this installs the tools of the psychophysical induction in their memory banks.

All levels of hypnotherapists, from beginner to advanced, generally use induction enhancement tools, but experienced hypnotherapists occasionally find opportunities for using advanced methods of induction as well. As a result, efficiency and effectiveness in certain private sessions may be increased. As students of hypnotherapy gain more experience practicing hypnotherapy, they may notice opportunities to use advanced hypnotic inductions.

Chapter 10

Avoiding and Handling Resistance

Resistance has a broad spectrum of meaning. Hypnotherapists that cannot get a client under hypnosis will often claim that the client is resisting. If a therapist doesn't get the desired results with a client, resistance is often the reason why. Some believe there is no such thing as resistance, but that the therapist needs to be more flexible with the methods that he or she uses to create change. Some believe that incompetent therapists experience resistance. This leads us to our broad definition of resistance.

Definition of Resistance

Anything that stands in the way of intention and the manifestation of that intention.

Everybody with normal psychological and physiological functioning can undergo hypnosis. No normal person is insusceptible, unless he or she desires not to participate in the hypnosis activity. In that case, the person is resisting.

Common causes of resistance to hypnosis are often rooted in misconceptions. The best way to avoid resistance is to have a thorough client interview that includes steps designed to reveal and answer the client's concerns about undergoing hypnosis. This is considered to be a preventive technique, because if resistance is headed off in the beginning, it will not persist throughout the session.

Two ways to prevent resistance

1) Question & Answer List- Upon a client's entrance into a hypno-therapist's office, the client generally will pick up client interview forms from the receptionist. A reception table is a good alternative, if a receptionist is absent and there is a sign asking clients to fill out the interview forms on the table. In either case, next to the interview forms can be another form which lists the most common questions asked and answered regarding hypnosis and hypnotherapy (refer to the chapter, Misconceptions of Hypnosis, to view this form).

2) Key Questions- There are two key questions that will reveal mis-conceptions with or without the use of a question-answer list:

a) "What concerns do you have about hypnosis?"
This question presupposes that the client has concerns about hypnosis, so that if they do exist, the client will reveal them. Upon revealing the concerns, the hypnotherapist needs only answer these and not those that are generalized from other clients. This approach can save time with handling only the individual misconceptions when they exist.

b) "What is your exposure to hypnosis?"
This question presupposes that the client has been exposed to hypnosis in some way, which is true in every case or the client would not have made it as far as to have made the appointment. In other words, the client has seen hypnosis on television, his or her mother had used it for anesthesia during childbirth when the client was born, or perhaps the client heard about it through a friend. They have been exposed to it in some way, and if it was a positive exposure, the hypnotherapist can direct the session to the

next step. If it has not been a positive exposure, such as watching the entertainment hypnosis on television, then there should be a short period of time spent answering a misconception and thereby putting fears to rest.

It is important to remember that in many cases, there are no concerns about trying hypnosis, so we do not want to create them by focusing on misconceptions that do not exist. Many times, client and therapist can simply proceed to the next step, without discussing misconceptions.

Below are the most common reasons for clients resisting hypnosis and hypnotherapy:

Reasons for Resistance:
1. Extreme tension and anxiety
2. The client wants to observe and not participate
3. The client is feeling self conscious
4. The client is over analytical
5. The client is trying too hard
6. The hypnotherapist's voice and presentation are disturbing
7. Lack of rapport
8. Fear of symptom removal

1) Extreme tension and anxiety:
        If there is a lot of anxiety in a client's life at the time a hypnotherapy session is given, the client may have an inability to focus his or her attention on that which is being suggested, particularly if those stresses are not related to the goal of hypnotherapy. Another tension may exist when a client has a stressful event occur immediately before the session (e.g. the client may have had a fender-bender on the way to the hypnotherapist's office). There are multiple reasons for tension and anxiety, and because hypnosis involves states of relaxation, it is best to attempt to resolve these before hypnosis is applied.

2) The client wants to observe and not participate:

Sometimes clients are focused on what the hypnotherapist is doing, rather than experiencing the suggestions given them. They may play the role of a private investigator while the hypnotherapist attempts relaxation exercises. Often, these clients peer through a crack in their eye lids to see what the hypnotherapist is doing. Sometimes they fidget in the trance chair.

3) The client is feeling self conscious:

Some clients wonder what they look like with their eyes closed or what the hypnotherapist may be observing about them. Some feel vulnerable with their eyes closed laying or sitting there in front of a complete stranger, or somebody they have only known for thirty to sixty minutes.

4) The client is over-analytical:

Some people tend to observe the process too much. Most of these people are left brain dominant. These personalities try to make sense of the suggestions, or analyze them, rather that just imagining and internalizing them. Those who fall into this category may still be able to undergo hypnosis with some instruction of how to engage in right brain imagery exercises; however, their experience is often less profound, and sometimes of a lighter trance level, when compared to the experiences of right brain dominant individuals.

5) The client is trying too hard:

Every once in a while, a hypnotherapy client will talk about how hard he or she tried to relax and imagine the suggestions given. This is more often the case when listening to self-hypnosis tapes. It occurs because the client is anxious to receive the benefits of hypnotherapy. Hypnosis is a predominantly right brain activity, involving simply imagining impressions. "Trying" is a left brain activity, and it can prevent relaxation, which is required at some level to achieve concentration and hypnosis. Worries over succeeding with the relaxation exercises given for induction increases stress and prevents hypnosis.

6) The hypnotherapist's voice and presentation are disturbing:

In some cases, the hypnotherapist's voice may be perceived as disturbing. Sometimes, even with a good "trance voice," as I refer to it, there is still a problem with the client's preferences in voice tonality or patter. Some clients have had unpleasant experiences with people who have certain voice qualities, and the hypnotherapist's voice and mannerisms may remind them of that problematic person from the past. In some cases, the voice of the hypnotherapist is too nasally or loud.

7) Lack of rapport:

Rapport is a necessary step in order to achieve success. Without rapport, there is a lack of trust. Without trust on the part of the client, it is very difficult to suggest any idea with a sufficient level of credibility. Most researchers in the field of clinical hypnosis believe that it is the most important factor in achieving a successful trance induction (read more about rapport in the chapter, Client Interview).

8) Fear of symptom removal:

Some clients desire change, but they have a fear of giving up a problem that has become a comfortable habit. Often, problematic habitual behaviors have secondary gains, which may not have been addressed in the client interview. When these are addressed, clients should be challenged with how they will continue to fulfill these secondary gains, or needs, that the problem was providing them. In cases of habit cessation, there is often an anxiety over giving up something he or she will miss and there is a fear of deprivation. Most clients have this anxiety at the beginning of the first office visit, but it rarely persist after clients are hypnotized and suggestions are given toward resolving the problematic goal.

Ways to Handle Resistance

On rare occasions, even after discussing misconceptions and expectations, resistance is still encountered. When it is, there are ways to handle resistance that can increase a person's success in achieving hypnosis and hypnotherapeutic results. The primary ways that this is achieved, in general, is to...*utilize the resistant behavior for the development of hypnosis.* If a hypnotherapist remembers this one concept, there will be many ways that he or she can accomplish this on a spontaneous basis, creating tools and techniques for handling resistance during the process of providing a hypnotherapy session.

Below are some good techniques I have used over the years that fall under the category of utilizing the behavior for the development of hypnosis:

A) If a client keeps opening his or her eyes, it can be suggested, "You can keep opening your eyes, but it's easier to concentrate on my suggestions with your eyes closed, so each time you open and close them, you will go deeper." This is known as a deepening technique called "compound suggestion," which will be explained in the chapter on deepening techniques.

B) If a client seems to question a lot of things, is over rationalizing the process, or seems left brain dominant, the hypnotherapist can suggest, "Now we're going to let the conscious mind do what it wants, to rationalize, analyze, and make decisions, but we're also going to let the subconscious mind do what it wants to do, which is to imagine the things that I am saying. So let's have the conscious rational self move aside, doing what it wants to off to the side, and let the subconscious mind imagine all of these relaxing ideas at the same time."

C) If a client is accustomed to a specific method of relaxation, like meditation, or a specific hypnotic induction he or she was hypnotized with in the past, the hypnotherapist can ask him or her specifics, (e.g. "What was it that really worked well for you to help you relax in the past.") Some clients will have had successful hypnosis methods that they will describe, others may describe a favorite vacation or other image, which can be reproduced for success. Most clients will give the hypnotherapist an example of some type of successful process of relaxation. In rare cases, some people will not have a clue of what it will take to help them relax.

In these cases, patience and perseverance with the use of a variety
of induction tools will be the key to success.

Common Causes of Resistance

Generally, resistance is a result of three primary areas:

1) Unresolved fears and misconceptions
2) Overuse of the conscious mind
3) A lack of rapport.

These may discovered somewhere in the middle of a hypnosis session, and it is at that point that the hypnotherapist must
"think on their feet" and come up with a positive and productive
concept that will propel them and their clients forward into getting results. Responding to clients from where they are within
themselves is the key to moving beyond the resistances that may
occasionally surface during hypnotherapy sessions. Exercising
patience is the key to getting past resistance.

Fortunately, resistance is encountered only in a minority of
instances. The majority of the time, particularly with broad spectrum inductions, such as the psychophysical inductions taught in
this book, people undergo hypnosis rather easily.

Chapter 11

Deepening Techniques

Twenty percent of the population is susceptible to a quick-deep trance level. Often this occurs at the very start of a hypnotic induction. These clients are referred to as being *Somnambulistic,* or *somnabulists*. These clinical hypnosis terms are not to be confused with the psychological term "somnambulism," which refers to a sleep disorder. Over a period of time, anyone who practices forms of hypnosis on themselves, such as self-hypnosis or meditation, has a higher chance of becoming somnambulistic.

Arons claimed that the deepest level of hypnosis was achieved in six to ten sessions, while Milton Erickson cited a positive correlation between the frequency that a client underwent hypnosis and the depth level that he or she achieved. Dave Elman wrote that the deepest level of hypnosis occurred on the fifth hypnotic induction. If we take these researchers' findings into consideration, we can predict that the more times a person undergoes an altered state of conscious, the deeper will be the state achieved.

What follows is a list of deepening techniques with scripts that give the hypnotherapist an idea of how to apply them with proper wording. Each has been designed to relax the mind and body in a more rapid and profound manner. They also indicate movement, implying that a client is traveling from one form of consciousness into another, and most involve imagery. It is recommended that two or three deepening techniques be used in combination with a hypnotic induction, as that would allow most clients to be deep enough to achieve effective therapeutic results. These are very powerful tools and should only be used by the trained professional hypnotherapist.

Deepening Techniques

1) Counting Techniques:

a) Numbers- This technique involves the hypnotherapist counting numbers aloud from one to five, or one to ten. Usually, the subject is told that they will be reaching their deepest level at the last number in the sequence. Hypnotherapists will tell their clients that they will go ten times, one hundred times, or perhaps one thousand times deeper with each number.

Numbers Script- "OK now, when I count from one to ten, you will go one thousand times deeper; one hundred times deeper with each number you hear without even trying. One, and one hundred times deeper. Two, two hundred. Three...farther. Four... four hundred. Five...deeper. Six...(pause) Seven....and seven hundred. Eight...deeper. Nine...(pause) and Ten... one thousand times more deeply relaxed."

b) Scales- The most common scale used for deepening is a yard stick. Because some people grew up with unpleasant disciplinary experiences, I have found the inclusion of the protective suggestion "a yardstick of your favorite color" to bring favorable results. The individual is told that thirty-six is the lightest level of trance, and inch number one is the deepest. The next time the hypnotherapist says the word "slide," the client is instructed to move down toward the number one, the deepest level of hypnosis.

Scales (Yard stick) Script- "I want you to imagine a yardstick with your favorite color. Inch number thirty six represents your lightest state of relaxation and inch number one is the deepest. The next time I say the word "slide," I want you to go down toward the number one, your deepest level. Slide down now to the number one. Slide all the way down. Slide down, very deep."

2) Ideomotor Techniques:

a) Breathing- Everyone must breathe to live, so this particular technique is very natural and effective. In addition, deep breathing is automatically a form of relaxation on its own. The client is simply instructed that he or she will go into a deeper trance level with each breath taken.

Breathing Script- "...and now with each breath that you take, allow yourself to become more deeply relaxed...simply deeper with each breath...inhaling the light of relaxation and exhaling any tensions or tightness so that you may go deeper, (pause), deeper, (pause), and even deeper.

b) Finger Signal- Clients are told to put themselves into their deepest state of relaxation within the next few minutes, and when they reach that level, they are asked to raise their index finger on one hand to indicate entering into their deepest level of hypnosis. Generally, the hypnotherapist automatically combines the Pause Technique below with this one, waiting for the finger to raise during the pause. Some people feel their finger raise subconsciously without effort, while others feel it shake or flicker, and then intentionally raise it with some conscious effort. One primary advantage of this particular technique is that it requires less effort on the part of the hypnotherapist as it transfers some of the responsibility for entering a deeper trance level to the client.

Finger Signal Script- "You know where your deepest level of relaxation is, so I will pause for a couple of minutes and you'll be able to go there automatically. You'll be able to raise your index finger when you get there. It may even flicker by itself to let you know you are at your deepest level...Go there now."

3) Pause Technique:

This tool has also been referred to as a *silence technique,* because the therapist is silent for a few minutes during a pause in speaking. Sometimes these pauses can be timed in a rhythmic fashion, such as at the end of each sentence when a breath is taken for the next sentence. This pausing effect can have a tendency to slow the speed of the client's breathing as well, as he or she begins to pace the hypnotherapist's breathing, deepening the trance with each pause.

Longer pauses can also be utilized, perhaps in conjunction with a finger signal. It is recommended that the hypnotherapist refrain from pausing more than a couple of minutes. Generally, pauses are effective from five seconds to one minute. Longer pauses may lose the attention of the client, and the activity of self-talk within the client's mind may take over, lightening the trance.

Pause Script- "I'm going to be silent for a minute. During that time, you can allow yourself to go much deeper into a state of relaxation, automatically, all on your own."

4) Scension Techniques:

a) Steps- The client is asked to imagine a "safe" flight of stairs, thereby avoiding the possibility of triggering an unpleasant memory of falling down stairs. It's advisable to refrain from describing the stairs as ascending or descending for the client, as some clients find it more relaxing to go up, while others prefer to go down. It is best to suggest that the stairs may be going *up or down,* and the client may choose which direction will take them deeper into hypnosis. I also like to combine this deepening technique with counting. I tell the client that there are ten stairs and at the tenth step, he or she will be at the deepest level of hypnosis.

Steps Script- "Imagine that there's a safe flight of stairs before you... ten stairs... I'm going to count from one to ten, and when I reach the number ten, you'll be at your deepest level of relaxation. Take the first step at One. Two, deeper. Three... Four, farther. Five... Six... Seven... Eight... Nine... Ten. Deeply Relaxed."

b) Elevators- The client is instructed that he or she is in a building of relaxation and that there are ten floors. The basement level is the deepest level. The client is to imagine that he or she is on the tenth floor and traveling down to the basement level. When the client arrives at the basement floor, the door opens and there is a hallway of light where he or she may proceed to someplace that is special or therapeutically valuable to them. Provided the client does not have claustrophobia, this technique is generally effective for deepening hypnosis.

Elevator Script- "Imagine that you are on the tenth floor of the building of relaxation. There's a safe elevator that can transport you to the basement level, which is the deepest level of relaxation.

The elevator doors open and you step onto it, press the "B" button, for basement, and it starts gradually descending. Deeper... deeper... and deeper, all the way down to the basement level. The doors open and there's a hallway that leads you..."

c) Escalators- This technique is very similar to the elevator exercise. The client is asked to take an escalator to a deeper level. Then, the client safely and comfortably steps onto the next floor or next depth level.

Escalator Script- "Imagine that there's an escalator before you. The escalator will take you to your deepest level of relaxation. As you step onto the escalator, it safely and comfortably takes you there now (long pause). And you get off at the next most deepest level."

d) Floating- It is suggested to the client to float to the place that represents the deepest level. He or she is told to float any direction that is necessary to get there. Abstract descriptions, such as "that place" were commonly and successfully used by Milton Erickson, because the unconscious mind would have to work to fill in the suggested image, deepening the trance. It is often best to combine counting from one to five with this technique. Floating is a kinesthetically dominant technique, which most clients can relate to and accomplish.

Floating Script- "Imagine that you are floating toward your deepest level. Because you know where that deepest level is, you will simply feel yourself float there when I count from one to five. One, floating. Two, farther. Three, more relaxed. Four, deeper. And Five, deeply relaxed."

5) Confusion Techniques:

a) Fractionation- This technique is good when others have failed or we have a resistant client. By going in and out of hypnosis repetitively during the same hypnosis session, the client's conscious mind becomes confused, and he or she naturally goes deeper. However, clients often report a level of discomfort associated with this particular technique. One advantage that Dave Elman cited was that this technique, which he referred to as "compounding the suggestion,"[10] lessened the frequency to depth requirements, in order to reach the deepest level of hypnosis, from five sessions to one. In other words, by fractionating a client five times, the client goes as deep as if they had undergone five hypnotic inductions, the fifth one being the deepest level.

Fractionation Script- "I'm going to count back from three to one. When I reach the number one, you will briefly awaken, but when I snap my fingers like this (snap fingers), you will be able to close your eyes and go much deeper than before. *Again...I'm going to count back from three to one. When I reach the number one, you will briefly awaken, but when I snap my fingers like this (snap fingers), you will be able to close your eyes and go much deeper than before. Three, more in touch with the room around you now. Two, the mind and body are returning back toward normal. And one, open your eyes, just briefly open your eyes now and (snap fingers). Deeper, deeper, and even deeper than before. Farther... Deeper with each breath...(pause)." [Repeat this three to five times from the * sign above]

b) Ambiguity- This is where the hypnotherapist's voice and words become so ambiguous that the subject simply allows the conscious mind to release its lock on them, thus the activities of analyzing or rationalizing are subdued. This effect is accomplished by telling the client that while experiencing a state of hypnosis, he or she will be able to hear the words from time to time, but that sometimes they won't be audible. He or she will be able to let go of the need to hear them consciously. Instead, the subject's unconscious mind will absorb them without effort. From there, the hypnotherapist continues to make his or her words understandable, then mumbles them, then lowers the voice until reaching a garbled whispering, and then back up to an audible level again.

This pattern is repeated until the strain to hear on the part of the client is notably nonexistent, and a serene expression is reflected upon the face, as if letting go of the need to consciously listen to the words.

This technique is contraindicated for hearing impaired individuals, since they tend to be anxious about their ability to hear. However, it is an effective exercise for individuals with a strong left brain dominance or an overactive conscious mind.

Ambiguity Script- "What will happen from here is that my voice will get louder and then softer, and sometimes you won't be able to understand the words consciously, but your subconscious mind will absorb them any way. It will understand the words without even trying, automatically. Your conscious mind will sometimes hear the words, and sometimes it won't. So now you can go deeper with each breath, automatically, you're going deeper and... so... its... yes... and that's... because there's deep.... relaxa... (mumbling softly)... deep... slee... farth... (now speak slightly louder) as you feel the body rest deeply, simply letting go it falls loose and limp and the mind goes to that place of deep peace, farther, (mumbling softly), so that... and.. slee... relax... farther... and it even... yes... and that's how far... deeper.. (ramble and blend words together).

6) Reframing Techniques:

a) Conscious Mind- This tool is used for the left brain dominant client, or the type who over analyzes and rationalizes, indicated by fidgeting during the hypnosis session. As a result, the effect is one of conscious mind resistance. In other words, the client's subconscious mind is not receiving the words on an impressionistic level, so his or her imagination is engaged. Instead, the conscious mind is intercepting practically every word that the hypnotherapist is suggesting and rationalizing it away. Once a hypnotherapist observes this, or is informed of this by the client, he or she may acknowledge that this effect is present and allow it by mentioning that this personality characteristic is natural for the client. As with all resistance, it is important to utilize it for the development of hypnosis.

The hypnotherapist may explain that this rational activity can continue to take place during the session, but that it will take a back seat to the subconscious mind's desire to equally imagine everything that is suggested. Another reframe is to suggest that most of the rational mind's activity of deciding whether or not hypnosis is working will be saved for later, after the session is done. The client's conscious mind can make sense of it at the end of the session and allow the subconscious mind to participate in imagining all of the relaxing ideas mentioned, for now.

Reframing The Conscious Mind Script- "Now the conscious mind needs to be acknowledged for its wonderful ability to rationalize, analyze, and make decisions about what's happening, but we're going to ask it to do these things later. We're asking it to wait until after the session to do these things, so that the subconscious mind can still receive suggestions in the form of images. It's going to move aside now, so that the subconscious is able to imagine things. Even if it seems like it's making it up, the subconscious mind's job is to imagine in the form of pictures, sounds, and feelings. The conscious mind can simply move aside and do its thing, while the subconscious can do its natural thing of simply just imagining things."

b) Depth (double bind)- Often, clients question at what point they will begin to experience a sufficient depth level for hypnotherapy to be effective. As a result, the hypnotherapist may give the client the suggestion that he or she will experience his or her deepest trance level right now, or wait to go there within the next two minutes, and then proceed with a deepening exercise. This has been referred to as a "double bind" hypnotic language pattern by those who have studied the hypnosis arts of Milton Erickson. It puts the unconscious mind in a double bind, so that an individual may choose one or the other, thus the individual goes to his or her deepest level now, or within the next two minutes. The mind generally needs alternatives when making decisions, and the therapist is providing alternatives that influence the client to enter into a win/win experience.

Double Bind Script- "You have a choice to either go to your deepest level right now, or you could wait just a few minutes until the end of this exercise to do so. Either way, you are going to go to your deepest level of relaxation. Remember what it feels like to be very, very deeply relaxed. Remember a time when the body was very tired at the end of the day and you laid down and let it just melt into the pads that you were laying against, as all the muscles relaxed at once, totally relaxing and content to be relaxing that deeply. And your mind just wanted to let go, completely. So you let it wander into a deep, distant direction, of deep, deep sleep (pause). Imagine that deep, deep, state of relaxation for the next few moments."

7) Rehearsal Technique:

a) Sleep- This word is often taken out of context and misunderstood, therefore causing misconceptions that hypnosis *is* sleep. However, when the word "sleep" is used by a hypnotherapist to deepen the trance, the subject already knows of the deep levels of relaxation that exist having experienced natural sleep. As a result, the subject can rehearse sleep and achieve a much deeper state of hypnosis. Therefore, this technique is generally very effective, provided the subject understands that he or she is to rehearse sleep, experiencing the relaxation effects of sleep, and not experiencing the actual sleep state itself. In order to avoid misconceptions, a protective suggestion I recommend hypnotherapists use would be that the word "sleep" is a suggestion to have the client relax to a similar depth level to natural sleep.

b) Unconsciousness- The word "unconsciousness" is also a rehearsal technique similar to the word "sleep." It is simply another state of mind signifying deep relaxation. Therefore, rehearsing this state may bring about the subjective experience of being void of conscious thoughts for a period of time. This experience is similar to that which many proficient meditators are able to produce... the "blank mind" effect. Because many people have had unpleasant states of unconsciousness, however, (chemoanesthesia, etc.) it is best to include the protective suggestion of a "pleasant unconsciousness." The script below incorporates both rehearsal techniques.

Rehearsal Script- "When I say the word 'sleep,' it simply means that you imagine what it would be like to become so relaxed that you experience a relaxation level that is as deep as the sleep state. Imagine what it would be like to be asleep. So sleep now. Sleep... Sleep... Deeper, asleep. Sleep... Sleep. Imagine a pleasant unconsciousness where there are no thoughts, now. A pleasant unconsciousness... Unconsciousness... deeper, into, unconsciousness... Unconsciousness... Sleep... Sleep."

When the subconscious mind has its own agenda...

A unique aspect of using deepening techniques to achieve a deep level trance is how the subconscious mind becomes more active in spontaneously selecting a therapeutic goal. Sometimes, the subconscious mind has its own agenda, regardless of the conscious goal set up at the beginning of the session, and a client's subconscious mind will select something to work on automatically. Because the *subconscious mind always selects the most important information at the time*, it is best to trust the subconscious mind's selection.

For example, I remember when a student took me down a flight of stairs during the deepening technique instructional part of my entry level hypnotherapy certification course. As she began to count me down the steps, I had a memory of when I was five years old and fell down the steps, hitting my head very hard against the basement floor. As the student observed my head rolling around on my shoulders and my face displaying abreaction, she became concerned because this was obviously not the intended experience. After the session, I assured her that my subconscious mind selected the most important information for me to experience at that time. Nonetheless, the session revolved around the fall rather than a simple deepening technique, which was unintentional.

Due to the fact that deepening techniques pacify or slow the activities of the conscious mind, occasionally an abreaction will surface from the unconscious mind. Because these memories or images can surface spontaneously, the hypnotherapist would want to be prepared to handle these experiences with patience, and not overreact. Even if a hypnotherapist is planning on specializing and only working with suggestive therapy, a client may still have negative memories surface spontaneously, particularly when in a deeper level trance.

One tool used to avoid this occasional effect is to suggest to the client that "the memory will fade away now like a dream" and they will temporarily forget about it, immediately refocusing their attention to another subject matter. On the other hand, if the therapist is trained in regression therapy, he or she may work the client through the memory images and help him or her obtain a therapeutic benefit.

If a hypnotherapist plans on using deepening techniques, he or she will experience more profound results. Clients feel a deeper sense of relaxation and often appreciate that they have undergone a detectable state of hypnosis, expecting that they will get better results. Sometimes, clients go so deep that they go somnambulistic and automatically forget what happened during hypnosis. Sometimes, they pass from hypnosis into sleep, such as some cases of suggestive therapy using scripts. Yet, the suggestions still get absorbed subconsciously and therapeutic results transpire.

Sometimes, clients go too deep for regression. They are simply too detached from the present environment. In this case, it is best to bring the client out of hypnosis a bit, lightening the trance. This can be done by asking the client to become more aware of the present moment and the room that he or she is in. Then, the question may be asked, "Can you talk to me now?" Once a verbal response is achieved, as opposed to a moan or groan, a regression method can be attempted again.

For most applications, deepening techniques make hypnotherapy more effective and create more successful outcomes. Profound states of consciousness result that are often exciting for client and hypnotherapist.

Chapter 12

Signs Of Hypnosis

Signs of hypnosis are indicators that prove to a client or hypnotherapist that a client has undergone a state of hypnosis. They involve physiological and psychological measurements. These two primary categories for signs of hypnosis are further explained as follows:

1) Physiological signs- These signs can be observed while a client is under hypnosis, so they are generally considered as objective measurements. They are generally physical involuntary responses. Direct observation of these signs can result in the accurate assumption by a hypnotherapist that a client is under a state of hypnosis.

2) Psychological signs- These are subjective measurements whereby the hypnotized individual will report specific experiences that are unusual, in comparison to his or her normal waking state. Though these signs are probably somehow connected to the physiological signs, they are not able to be observed by the practicing hypnotherapist. They are part of the client's mental awareness and therefore only recognized when the client reports his or her mental perceptions of the hypnotic experience.

Many individuals who desire the results hypnotherapy offers also want *proof* that something has transpired which will lead to change. The signs of hypnosis tend convince both client and hypnotherapist that a client has experienced an adequate state of hypnosis. In a high majority of cases, when individuals undergo a state of hypnosis, they experience one or more of the signs listed below.

Physiological Signs:
a. Eye lids tremble or flutter when closed (R.E.M.)
b. Eyes become glassy and red, a fixed stare when open
c. Actions slow or cease for long periods of time
d. Limp facial muscles, expressionless
e. Pause before responses
f. Speech is quiet, slowed, or slurred
g. Excessive salivation and swallowing
h. Slowed respiration
i. Slowed heart rate
j. Increased galvanic skin response
k. Decrease in metabolism
l. Decrease in blood pressure
m. Predominant alpha and theta brain-wave patterns
n. Involuntary physical movements

Psychological Signs:
a. Enhanced memory capabilities
b. Feelings of peacefulness and calmness
c. Sensations of extreme heaviness
d. Feeling immobile
e. Sensations of floating or weightlessness
f. Tingling sensations in the hands or feet
g. Hyper-awareness (all five senses awakened)
h. Enhanced imagery capability
i. Feeling a sense of detachment (dissociation)
j. Time distortion—underestimating or overestimating time
k. Spontaneous psychological manifestations
l. Disinclination toward awakening
m. Feelings of numbness
Physiological Signs of Hypnosis

a. Eye lids tremble or flutter when closed (R.E.M.)

Often, individuals will start experiencing rapid eye movement at the start of the induction. This movement tends to be very rapid in the lighter, alpha state. The observer will notice the eyes moving more slowly, back and forth from side to side, as the state of hypnosis deepens.

b. Eyes become glassy and red, a fixed stare when open

If the client opens his or her eyes during hypnosis or after being awakened, the eyes will appear to be red, teary, or glassy. This is likely due to the change in blood pressure, which also occurs during normal sleep states. This effect may also be due to rapid eye movements.

c. Actions slow or cease for long periods of time

Because the state of hypnosis lies between the states of awake and asleep, there is a disinclination toward movement, particularly in the deeper levels of hypnosis. This effect is a sign that an individual is experiencing alpha or theta brain waves.

d. Limp facial muscles, expressionless

The observer will notice a serene look upon the client's face. This is a limp-expressionless look, due to a deep level of relaxation in the facial muscles.

e. Pause before responses

This effect occurs primarily while conducting a hypnotic regression. When the hypnotherapist asks the client a question for the purpose of finding out what the subject is experiencing, there tends to be a long pause before response. This is because hypnosis slows down the conscious mind to an extent that it generally operates about four times slower than it does in the normal waking state.

f. Speech is quiet, slowed, or slurred

This effect is also because of altered state brain waves, causing the body to respond in a lethargic fashion. It may be similar to a person just awakening from sleep in the morning when they are not yet fully awake.

g. *Excessive salivation and swallowing*

This experience may be observed only in the minority of individuals who undergo hypnosis. It is not thoroughly researched and understood as to the reasons why this effect exists.

h. *Slowed respiration*

This effect may be researched in many written clinical resources referring to altered states. Various forms of relaxation lead to slowed breathing rates which may easily be observed in hypnotized subjects.

i. *Slowed heart rate*

This effect is a result of undergoing an altered state or alpha and theta brain waves. It is not easily observable without measurement devises. However, Milton Erickson had been known to detect the pulse of some of his clients through the visual inspection of their throat or ankle.

j. *Galvanic skin response*

This response indicates sympathetic nervous system involvement which increases with emotional excitement. Fluctuations in the skin's electrical resistance is a result of sweat gland activity.

k. *Decrease in metabolism*

This effect is created from any altered state, particularly hypnosis. It is positively correlated with levels of relaxation. Deep sleep creates the slowest metabolism.

l. *Decrease in blood pressure*

This effect is created from any form of relaxation, particularly hypnosis. As a result, stress and hypertension may be reduced or eliminated through a daily regiment of self-hypnosis.

m. *Predominant alpha and theta brain-wave patterns*

It has been proven in various hypnosis research texts that hypnosis is characterized by alpha and theta brain wave patterns.

These indicate light to deeper levels of hypnosis respectively. (See chapter on depth correlations.)

n. Involuntary physical movements
Sometimes clients will experience the twitching of a limb, finger, or facial muscle. Sometimes these are due to memories experienced under hypnosis, but sometimes they spontaneously occur for no significant reason. These can be embarrassing to the client, but it is best to ignore their presence, unless the client mentions them.

Psychological Signs of Hypnosis

a. Enhanced memory capabilities
Many individuals are not convinced that they have been under hypnosis, until they have experienced remembering information that they could not have remembered while in the normal beta-waking state. Clients who experience *hypermnesia*, or enhanced memories capabilities under hypnosis, usually will experience it through a hypnotic regression technique. However, sometimes clients do it spontaneously while under hypnosis. This is why every hypnotherapist should be trained in basic hypnotic regression and thereby recognize when memories under hypnosis occur spontaneously.

b. Feelings of peacefulness and calmness
Many people have never experienced such a peaceful-conscious form of relaxation as that of hypnosis. Most people enjoy this level of peace and calmness so much, that once they experience it, they desire to learn it and provide it for themselves on a regular basis. This effect generally improves a person's health and psychological disposition.

c. Sensations of extreme heaviness
Upon awakening from hypnosis, many have reported that they felt like "a ton of bricks," or like they "weighed a thousand

pounds." They report that their bodies felt as though they were asleep while their minds were aware of everything.

d. Feeling immobile
Some claim that they couldn't have moved their arms and feet even if they had tried. This can be a result of full body catalepsy, or deep trance phenomena. Yet, if there were an emergency, as deemed by the subject, he or she would be able to awaken themselves from hypnosis and respond to the situation at hand.

e. Sensations of floating or weightlessness
I remember a nurse who awoke from hypnosis and upon my asking about her experience told me, "Wow, that was so cool. I was starting to feel like I was floating, then I drifted up and started soaring (with excited hand gestures)." This case exemplifies how dramatic this sign actually becomes for some clients subjectively.

f. Tingling sensations in the hands or feet
It is speculated that this sensation is due to a change in the galvanic skin response. Some hypnotized subjects will claim that there is a numb feeling associated with a tingling sensation.

g. Hyper-awareness (all five senses awakened)
Many hypnotized individuals expect to become unaware of their surroundings. Yet, in the lighter to medium levels of hypnosis, there is the common experience of being hyper-aware of everything in a person's surroundings as well as within his or her mind's eye. The five sensory channels within the mind's eye (see, hear, feel, taste, and smell) become distinctly acute, therefore, imagery is clearer. This effect is called *hyperesthesia*. Everything the client perceives in his or her environment, while under hypnosis, becomes amplified by the senses. This occurs so much so that individuals under hypnosis can perceive this phenomenon as a distraction, yet if it weren't present, the next sign (enhanced imagery) would not be possible. It has been concluded by some hypnosis researchers that while an individual is in the waking state, he or she is aware of one to three things at a time; but while

an individual is in the hypnotic state, he or she is aware of seven to nine things at a time.

h. Enhanced imagery capability

Whatever a hypnotized person focuses on becomes amplified, because hypnosis magnifies every thought and experience. This magnifying effect is one of the greatest assets of hypnosis for creating change. Through hypnotic suggestion, clients can live the future before it takes place using future-based imagery, which becomes a future memory—one that is just as significant as any other memory.

i. Feeling a sense of detachment (dissociation)

There is a positive correlation with hypnotic depth and dissociation. The deeper an individual goes into hypnosis, the more detachment he or she experiences. Dissociating an individual can also deepen the trance level, such as the detachment that is often experienced during an induction. This occurs at the moment the hypnotherapist suggests imagery that directs a person's attention to a beautiful and relaxing place, such as the beach or mountains. As the induction proceeds, an individual becomes more and more dissociated from his or her immediate environment.

j. Time distortion (underestimating or overestimating time)

Time distortion is very common at any hypnotic level. Often, individuals who have undergone hypnosis will report that they feel that they have only been under hypnosis for fifteen minutes, when it's actually been forty five. Sometimes, individuals will report that they feel that they have been under hypnosis for an hour, when it's actually been twenty minutes. It is seldom that an individual reports the accurate transpiring of time. Perhaps it is because we actually are spiritual beings and hypnosis releases a person's consciousness from the physical-material world. Perhaps it is a mild form of the out-of-body phenomena that are often reported in our era.

k. Spontaneous psychological manifestations

Sometimes a person's mind will tend to wander into new dimensional realities, or foreign images. Everything from being aware of another place where people are riding bicycles to that of a dark dungeon have been reported. Sometimes these spontaneous images are pleasant to the client, and sometimes they are unpleasant. Sometimes they contain important character traits of the client, and they can be used as a form of therapy. Some clients report that they feel as if they have visited another place which was occurring in the present moment at the same time.

l. Disinclination toward awakening

For some hypnotized people, this effect is similar to that of waking up from normal sleep the first thing in the morning, when sometimes there is a tendency for an individual to avoid getting out of bed. The client often enjoys the sense of peace that hypnosis provides to the extent that there is a disinclination toward awakening. If clients avoid the awakening procedures, it is recommended that hypnotherapists take the steps to awaken them which are mentioned earlier in this book.

m. Feelings of numbness

There is a positive correlation between depth and anesthesia, so the deeper the state of hypnosis an individual achieves, the more numb he or she becomes. The numbness will often start in the hands and feet, then spread into the rest of the body. It is as if the body goes to sleep as the mind remains alert. Many surgeries have been performed by simply using a good subject who can maintain a deep state of hypnosis.

Using Signs as Convincers and Indirect Suggestions

Often, that which clients describe as their experience under hypnosis upon awakening can further convince them that they have undergone a state of hypnosis, thereby improving their results. For example, if a client awakens and the hypnotherapist asks them, "How do you feel?" the response will often include one or more of the signs of hypnosis, such as, "Wow, it felt like I was so heavy that I couldn't move." At that time the therapist could give the indirect suggestion as follows, "Well that's a sure sign that you've undergone a deep level of hypnosis, so you should get some nice results." This statement is actually true, because a deeper state of hypnosis had actually been achieved. In the chapter on suggestion, we will recognize that the deeper states of hypnosis ensure the acceptance of suggestion. In addition, when an individual undergoes hypnosis and reports or shows some of the signs, the results are automatically enhanced, because of the increase in the faith factor. Also, an indirect suggestion given at the time when a client's subconscious mind is still susceptible, when a client is awakening from hypnosis, increases therapeutic effectiveness. It is like putting the icing on the cake, metaphorically speaking.

Milton Erickson believed that every part of the session, the interview and post interview stages, left the client open to suggestion. In other words, clients tend to hang on every word that the therapist speaks as having significant meaning. Those researchers who have studied Erickson's work and written on their findings have referred to this process as utilizing indirect suggestions. These were often given when the client was out of traditional trance, but still open to influence. Erickson was a master at creating the most effective indirect suggestions for specific clients on-the-fly, or in a very spontaneous fashion. Once again, *creativity is a hypnotherapist's greatest asset*. Opportunities present themselves in the interview stages, and the signs of hypnosis are some of the easiest convincers, particularly utilized in combination with indirect suggestions.

The practitioner may choose to utilize his or her creative skills at certain key points during the client interview and post session interview.

Everybody is creative, to some extent. The process of creativity is similar to the first time we rode a bike. We began to create a balance. That balance wasn't achieved until we got onto the bike and started riding. That's when it started happening. We were forced to create at that one most significant moment by correcting or turning into balance. After that, all we had to do was turn the front wheel the right way and we automatically felt the balance again.

That's how practicing hypnotherapy is. The therapist and client both know when they have that balance, when they are doing "the dance," as I sometimes refer. Rapport, a type of inner knowingness, becomes present sometime during the therapeutic session, and the only way to experience it is to submit to the process. Rapport, what I sometimes refer to as, "sharing the same space," increases the chances for success.

Welcome to *indirect suggestion*. I just started off with something that was true and added other truths to it, then interwove it with a universal metaphor (the first bike ride) with the intent to influence readers to trust the process of creativity within sessions by submitting to experiential learning. The best part of all of it is that I believe everything I just described, and most will also find it to be true. As we shall see in the chapter that describes the laws of suggestion, truth lasts much longer than hallucination. In fact, truth will last a lifetime for most individuals.

Indirect suggestions are happening at all times during a client session, and they are most effective when we've established rapport. Practitioners should watch for opportunities to create these moments.

In summary, signs are indicators when observed. They tell hypnotherapists what level of hypnosis clients are in, or at least that the client is in a state of hypnosis. In addition, they provide opportunities to increase expectation toward achieving results, which can lead to greater levels of success.

Chapter 13

Depth Correlations and Phenomena

It is important for the hypnotherapist to consider which approach he or she is going to take, a research or a therapeutic approach. If an individual is taking the research approach, he or she may be able to hook the client up to an electroencephalogram (E.E.G.), which measures the brain waves of the client, and thereby objectively observe the depth of hypnosis. However, if the practicing hypnotherapist were to do this with his or her clients, it is likely that he or she may lose a lot of clients, due to the impersonality of this approach. It is only natural that hypnosis clients desire empathy, or a feeling that they are being understood. Machines often signify a lack of compassion, yet, it remains somewhat important for the hypnotherapist to get an idea of the depth of hypnosis that the client is experiencing.

As an alternative, through careful observation, subjective measurement tools may help hypnotherapists determine the client's depth. For example, if the hypnotherapist notices the client's breathing change to a guttural draw, like a mild snore, then it would be natural to assume that the client is in a deep or somnambulistic state of hypnosis. The jaw dropping open would also indicate this.

Other subjective measurements listed in the previous chapter, which discuss the physical signs of hypnosis, are also helpful in determining when a state of hypnosis exists.

Objective Measurements

By examining the electroencephalogram which follows, it would be safe to say that hypnosis is generally characterized by *alpha and theta* brain waves, as is indicated by most research involving hypnotized individuals. However, Wilda B. Tanner,[11] a popular author on dreams, discovered some brain wave research (in the following illustration) showing some well practiced yogis could reach the delta brain wave level of the altered state.

Tanner's Electroencephalograph:

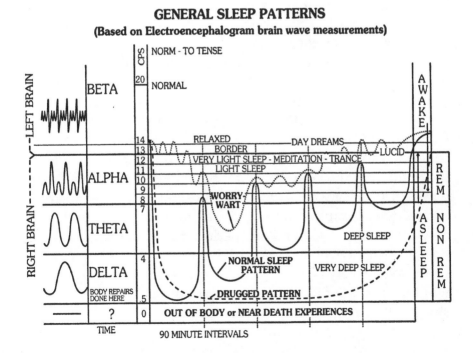

GENERAL SLEEP PATTERNS
(Based on Electroencephalogram brain wave measurements)

Just as in the rare case of one of these yogis, it is also quite possible that Edgar Cayce was able to induce a self-hypnotic trance to the level of delta, in order to accomplish his profound readings. Because there is a positive correlation between hypnotic amnesia and the depth of hypnosis, this may explain why Cayce often could not remember the things that he said upon his awakening from a state of hypnosis, and therefore he needed a person to record them, who was known as Gladys Davis.

Further examination of Tanner's E.E.G. shows that we experience the waking state while in beta brain waves, rapid eye movements (R.E.M.) while in alpha brain waves, and non-R.E.M. states in theta and delta. Because hypnosis is primarily a right brain activity, notice that the dividing line between alpha and beta is between 12 and 13 cycles per second (C.P.S.). This dividing line indicates an individual's natural ability to enter into hypnogogic states, such as daydreaming, from the normal waking state involving beta brain waves.

Research shows that the quickest way to increase alpha brain waves is to simply close the eyes. So automatically, at the beginning of the induction, when we request our clients close their eyes, we can assume that most individuals are going into a light state of hypnosis rather quickly.

Normal sleep cycles are indicated in Tanner's illustration as well. The sleep state is characterized by an individual completely losing conscious awareness in the deeper altered states of theta and delta brain waves. In normal sleep, the conscious mind detaches from the subconscious. In hypnosis, the conscious mind stays connected to the subconscious mind to transfer information, as the brain goes through alpha and theta brain waves. Delta brain waves virtually always characterize normal sleep. The illustration shows that we must enter into delta brain waves once or preferably twice each night or sleep period, for about 90 minutes at a time, in order to feel well rested. It is evident that individuals who worry excessively generally don't experience delta sleep, so they will not reap the full benefits of sleep, or obtain "a good night's sleep," often even feeling worse after sleeping.

Other areas of interest are the lucid dream areas, which are when we are aware that we are falling asleep, but remain awake at some level. This effect occurs at the 12/13 c.p.s. border. This area is where most people get very creative ideas. If creative people are not handling their stress levels well, they often will bypass this light alpha area when trying to relax to create. This is referred to as artist's block. The average person may recognize that this area, (just as he or she falls asleep or immediately awakens), is exactly where he or she will get his or her most creative ideas. For this reason, it is quite common for people to keep a pencil and paper next to their bed, in order to remember creative ideas and solutions to their problems.

The first popular individual in our history that recognized the beneficial aspect of a state of hypnosis involving its lucidity and creativity was Thomas Edison, inventor of the light bulb. He discovered that his most ingenious inventions came about when he was just crossing over into the altered state. As a result, he would try to reproduce this state and record the ideas that were encountered there. His method involved holding a metal ball, so that when he entered the level of relaxation indicative of the creative state, the metal ball would drop to the floor. Whatever he was thinking at that time, he generally placed importance upon and recorded. This is how he came up with the idea of the light bulb.

Another interesting portion of Tanner's illustration is that which Ms. Tanner found to be the areas correlating to "out of body" and "near death experiences" (O.O.B. and N.D.E. respectively). After researching these areas, she found that there was very little to no brain wave activity (0 to .5 C.P.S.) with those who have reported these experiences. These experiences are still being clinically researched for their authenticity, but some interesting data has come forward within the last decade. Many persons who have had this experience were able to document things that they said they had encountered while out of body, which they could not have possibly known unless they had visited there during the experience. One such book that speaks about an individuals experiences that may document this phenomena is *Saved By The Light,* by Danion Brinkley.

There are new discoveries concerning which parts of the brain show increased activity through glucose testing, or what is referred to within the field of neuroscience as brain tomography. By administering intravenous radioactive glucose to patients, brain researchers have discovered which areas of the brain are more active than others during specific activities. These areas simply use more glucose. These higher rates of glucose consumption show up on screen through Positron Emission Tomography (P.E.T.) scans and relative color coding. Through this research method, medical science has determined the activity of speech to be a left brain activity, because the brain consumes more glucose in the left brain hemisphere when an individual speaks. This same research indicates that hypnosis is generally a right brain activity, because this area of the brain usually uses more glucose during the altered state of hypnosis.

In Winifred Blake Lucas' book, *Regression Therapy: A Handbook For Professionals*, through what she called "mind mirroring," she hypothesized that different parts of the brain were in different brain waves during an altered state of consciousness. She theorized that part of the hypnotically regressed person's brain stayed in beta, and part in alpha or theta, in order to transfer the information from the subconscious to the conscious mind. This effect, as it is theorized, gives the client the ability to talk to the hypnotherapist while in a state of hypnosis.

According to brain researcher Richard M. Restak, M.D., in his artfully practical book, *The Brain*, we only use about 10% of our brain. This came about as a result of lesion testing. The first recognition that the brain was located in the head (and not the heart as previously thought), and that certain areas in the brain controlled specific areas of the body, was through ancient sword battles. When individuals were wounded with a cut in the back of the head, they would often become blind, because it produced damage in the occipital lobe, which is the part of the brain that is responsible for eyesight. Further research shows that regardless of how many lesions made in the brain, approximately 90% of these had no detectable effect on mental or physical functioning. Interestingly, most of the undetectable responses were lesions made in the areas of the brain known as "gray matter." Oddly enough, therefore, it was determined by neuroscientists and medical researchers that we humans only use about 10% of our brain.

Subjective Measurements

Below is a basic depth measurement scale. It is rather basic when considering other scales in other texts, but these classifications are adequate for understanding the use of hypnosis in therapy. For those desiring further research into other scales with several more subjective classifications, please refer to Masud Ansari's text, *Modern Hypnosis: Theory and Practice.*

Hypnotic Depth Scale:
1. Insusceptible
2. Hypnoidal / Hypnogogic
3. Light Trance
4. Medium Trance
5. Deep Trance / Somnambulistic
6. Sleep

Insusceptible simply means that an individual denies the suggestions to relax or is not concentrating on what the hypnotherapist is saying. In older texts, because of Freudian theories, the inadequacies brought about by the use of eye fixation, and limited education in hypnosis, it was claimed that some people were unable to undergo a state of hypnosis. Although this misconception continues to exist today, the fact is that every individual is able to undergo hypnosis, provided he or she has *normal physiological and psychological functioning*. However, from time to time, individuals simply choose not to participate in their imagination, and therefore do not enter into hypnosis.

Hypnoidal / Hypnogogic: Hypnoidal is a synonym of Hypnogogic; they have the same meaning. This trance level represents the every day lethargic state of mind. These states of mind are experienced automatically throughout a normal person's daily existence. States that signify this level include: daydreaming, highway hypnosis, watching an interesting television program, listening to a captivating story, repetitive movements (factory workers), and so on. This level of hypnosis is automatic and very natural. Hypnoidal level trances occur at the border of beta and alpha brain waves. Milton Erickson was the first to recognize the importance of the hypnogogic state and referred to this concept as "waking hypnosis."

Light Trance is achieved rather easily at the start of a hypnotic induction, or with a simple short induction. To ask an individual to close his or her eyes and imagine a restful scene enables this individual to achieve this level rather easily. An inner focus on the imagery process is often useful for obtaining this level, particularly with a progressive relaxation. This is all it takes for most individuals, however, somnambulists (those susceptible to a quick deep trance) may go much deeper than the average individual at the start of the induction. Light trance is beneficial for suggestive therapy and imagery based therapies, such as immune system therapy or nuerolinguistic programming. Light trance occurs in alpha brain waves.

Medium Trance is generally obtained with the use of a formal hypnotic induction. The formal induction involves a longer drawn-out induction mixing physically and mentally relaxing concepts. Medium level hypnosis is effective for performing regressions, as well as suggestive therapy sessions. Medium level trance occurs in the lower alpha or upper theta brain waves.

Deep Trance levels are experienced most often with individuals through a formal induction and at least two deepening techniques. If the individual is more left brain dominant, utilizing his or her conscious mind more, then he or she may need a longer induction with more deepening techniques, in order to achieve the deeper levels of trance. If the client is normal, or right brain dominant, then a couple of deepening techniques are certainly adequate. A sign of an individual experiencing a deep level of hypnosis is a guttural nose-throat sound, such as a mild snore. Loud snoring is a sure sign, but not the only indicator. Everyone can reach a deep level trance. Deep level trance is often referred to as *somnambulism*, which is defined as a *sleep-like state*. It occurs in the middle to deeper levels of theta brain waves.

Sleep occurs when an individual loses consciousness in a state of relaxation; in other words, an individual's conscious mind becomes detached from the present awareness. The conscious mind and the subconscious mind become one, as both experience the same thing. When individuals are in the sleep state, they could be asked a question and they would not be able to respond. Nonetheless, research shows that suggestions are often accepted by those that are in a state of sleep.

Hypnosleep

As long as the sleep state was entered while there was talking from an outside source, the sleeping individual's unconscious mind will be open to suggestion. During World War II, some American soldiers slept with a tape recorder under their pillow and found that there was a profound increase in their capability to learn the Japanese language. This is what I refer to as a form of *hypnosleep*. In addition, Dave Elman's book, *Hypnotherapy*, shows that he was able to produce hypnosleep, proving that individuals were able to unconsciously respond to questioning. This was done through an involuntary finger signaling method, whereby the person sleeping had their finger flicker as an indication of specific responses to certain questions.

I generally characterize hypnosleep as being a state that starts out with hypnosis and moves into the sleep state. This indicates that the hypnotized individual enters into sleep through another person's vocal direction, so the person remains open to suggestion. This effect occurs with self-hypnosis tapes, as individuals frequently fall asleep to these, yet gain the usual benefits of hypnosis. In rare cases, individuals have been known to be influenced with suggestion while sleeping, but the subjects had to have an aptitude toward the desired change, for such suggestions to have been effective.

The sleep state works just as well as traditional states of hypnosis for achieving successful suggestive therapy. However, if a hypnotherapist attempts regression and the subject falls asleep, it is going to be difficult or impossible to obtain a memory. The hypnotherapist needs to bring him or her into a lighter level in order obtain a regression...the place that is between awake and asleep. For this reason, a medium level of hypnosis, or at most—medium deep, is best for hypnotic regression.

Hypnotic Phenomena

Hypnotic phenomena is directly correlated with a person's level of trance. With this in mind, readers should be aware that light trance phenomena can equally occur in the medium and deep levels of trance, and medium trance phenomena can also occur in a deep trance. It is also important to keep in mind that no matter how deep the trance level, all of the laws of suggestion listed in the next chapter still apply, the most important involving clients' *willingness* to experience suggestions by using their imagination, in order for them to occur.

Light Trance Phenomena

a) <u>Eye Catalepsy-</u> The hypnotherapist tells the subject that the eyes are stuck closed. For a short period of time, he or she relaxes the eye muscles so much so that they feel stuck, and then the client is told to open them shortly thereafter.

b) <u>Arm Catalepsy-</u> The subject is told to hold out his or her arm and to imagine that the arm is a "bar of steel." When this happens in light trance, the arm goes rigid. When the subject is in a medium level of hypnosis, an unusual amount of weight may be supported by the arm, showing unusual strength.

c) <u>Kinesthetic Hallucinations-</u> These are the easiest to produce. Simply suggesting an itch while talking to someone in a normal waking state will produce scratching. How many people start checking themselves when someone finds a tick (a common parasite in the United States) on themselves? They often feel the crawling sensation even when there is nothing there. Emotions are easy kinesthetic hallucinations to produce. Suggesting something humorous generally triggers a laughter response in the lighter trance level, because individuals must relax in order to experience this emotion.

d) <u>Hyperesthesia-</u> This is where all five senses are awakened. Our visual, auditory, gustatory, olfactory, and kinesthetic sensory perceptual channels are supersensitive. Individuals are simultaneously aware of everything that is going on in the external environment, as well as within the mind's eye. This occurs in the light and medium depths of hypnosis, then, because of dissociation, it disappears when individuals are in a deep trance level.

Medium Trance Phenomena

a) <u>Memory Recall-</u> *Hypermnesia,* defined as enhanced memory capabilities, occurs with a medium state of hypnosis and is increased in the deeper level. When people recall a memory while they are under hypnosis, it becomes more clear when compared to a normal waking state. Memory recall is not as vivid as hypnotic age regression, however. Memory recall may be characterized as an experience of looking back at the past, rather than reliving it. In the lighter levels of hypnosis, an individual is able to recall a memory but he or she is somewhat dissociated from the memory and still more associated into the present moment. Medium levels of hypnosis enable a person to intermittently experience reliving the memory, or being more associated into it. At this level, talking in hypnosis occurs without awakening. However, since talking often can lighten a trance, it may be best to suggest to the subject that he or she will "be able to stay deeply relaxed and still be able to talk" to you. Medium levels of hypnosis are effective for both memory recall and age regression, but age regression is more consistent with deeper trance, while memory recall is associated with light to medium levels.

b) <u>Open Eyed Trance-</u> An individual doesn't have to have his or her eyes closed to experience hypnosis. Many subjects under hypnosis have opened their eyes while under hypnosis maintaining the ability to hallucinate and accept suggestions. In fact, if clients open their eyes while under hypnosis without being told that they are awakening, they will be fractionating themselves into a deeper trance level, which is also a traditional deepening technique commonly referred to as "fractionation."

c) <u>Olfactory Hallucinations</u>- In the medium level of hypnosis, an individual may smell things that do not actually exist in the environment. Research commonly suggests that the olfactory sense is directly associated with memory. Medium trance level characterizes this hallucination.

d) <u>Gustatory Hallucinations</u>- In the medium level of hypnosis, an individual may be able to taste something that is not present in the environment. A common stage hypnosis demonstration of this type of hallucination involves suggesting that an onion is really an apple and the volunteer should take a bite to enjoy the flavor. When an individual does so, he or she smiles and experiences the taste as an apple.

e) <u>Light Anesthesia</u>- In medium hypnosis, a level of anesthesia generally occurs that is adequate for most minor surgical procedures. It is best to use imagery with a medium trance level, to increase effectiveness. This combination is also generally effective for alleviating chronic pain.

f) <u>Time Distortion</u>- This effect is positively correlated with depth. It involves a client's estimation of the amount of time that he or she believes had transpired while under hypnosis. This time span is either grossly under estimated or over estimated.

g) <u>Dissociation</u>- This effect leads to the subject feeling detached from his or her immediate environment. This effect by itself is effective for producing hypnoanesthesia. It starts to occur in the induction during the imagery process, and it increases with trance depth. Individuals tend to experience this feeling of detachment while in a medium level of hypnosis.

Deep Trance Phenomena

a) <u>Age Regression-</u> In the deeper levels of trance, age regression with *revivification* takes place, which may be defined as reliving a memory or experience under hypnosis. The term, age regression, is associated with medium to deep level trances. Many describe this experience as having one foot in the present, and one foot in the past. Their five senses within the memory are very sharp, recalling names, dates, and places from adolescence, infancy, in-utero, and some believe from even past lifetimes. A deep trance level assists in assuring revivification, or in other words full memory association.

b) <u>Amnesia-</u> Amnesia is generally not possible without a deep level of hypnosis. It generally occurs spontaneously, but the hypnotherapist may suggest amnesia as well. As long as the subject is willing to forget an experience he or she had while under deep hypnosis *and* the hypnotherapist suggests it, this phenomenon can transpire effectively. If the subject denies the suggestion to forget, it will not work. Most individuals desire to remember what transpired under hypnosis, so they will automatically remember.

c) <u>Profound Anesthesia-</u> This effect is easily produced in somnambulists, who are those that undergo a quick deep trance rather easily. They must also be well practiced with the regular use of hypnosis. Profound anesthesia is effective for major surgeries, but the effect will wear off over a period of an hour or two. With the proper hypnosis candidate, and a surgery that will not last over a couple of hours, this technique can be as effective as chemoanesthesia. It is best that a hypnotherapist attend any major surgery, so that if the trance state lightens, it can be corrected with deepening techniques.

d) <u>Auditory Hallucinations-</u> To be able to hear something that does not exist in the external environment, an individual must have obtained a deep level trance. Auditory hallucinations, such as an individual hearing a ship's fog horn while he or she is participating in a hypnosis stage show at a hotel, are experienced most clearly with a deep trance level.

e) <u>Visual Hallucinations-</u> This effect requires a very deep trance, in order to be effectively produced and experienced. For example, seeing butterflies that are not in a person's immediate environment must occur as a result of being given such a suggestion while in a deep level trance. Somnambulists are the most likely to encounter visual hallucinations.

f) <u>Profound Dissociation-</u> This phenomenon is often experienced as a journey into another dimensional reality. Clients who experience this phenomenon often report feeling as if they had been transported to a place completely detached from the present moment. Upon awakening, some clients remember where their mind traveled to, and some do not, since they tend to have been in such a deep state of hypnosis, similar to a dream state. If they remember, it is there that they report many details, but because they are so detached from the hypnotherapist in the present moment, they tend to report these upon awakening.

For example, one individual who had an abstract regression, which is commonly referred to as a "past life regression," experienced being a Native American woman who was being drowned in a river by her tribe. Upon awakening from a deep level of hypnosis, she had rope burns left on her wrists from where she had been tied and led to the river. Like many who attempt abstract regression, she was left with a feeling that the memory was a true recount of her souls path, so the red marks that appeared for a short time served as the important proof that she desired.

During this phenomenon, an individual can feel like he or she is about 90 percent aware of another place or time, and only 10 percent aware of the present at the same time. However, it is important to understand that profound dissociation does not typically occur under regression; it tends to occur spontaneously and more often as a result of using a combination of suggestive and deepening techniques. Many people in hypnosis stage shows tent to experience this phenomena from having been fractionated. Additionally, both hypnoanesthesia and age regression are greatly enhanced when profound dissociation exists.

Hypnotic Hallucination

Positive hallucination involves the suggestion to add something to a person's awareness, such as suggesting there is a clock on the wall that is not in the external environment. *Negative hallucination* involves taking away something from the environment that is actually there, such as suggesting that an individual cannot see a clock that is actually hanging on a wall. *Delusion* involves changing a person's perception to reflect something different than what is actually present in the external environment. For example, a hypnotist may suggest that a clock reads twelve midnight, when in fact it reads three in the afternoon. Yet, the hypnotized individual experiences a tiredness that is associated with midnight.

The following is a rating of hypnotic hallucination from the easiest (light trance), at the top of the list, to most difficult (deep trance), at the bottom of the list:

Tactile hallucination
Olfactory hallucination
Gustatory hallucination
Auditory hallucination
Visual hallucination

Two Primary Hallucination Theories

There are two primary theories that I have created from years of research in the subject, in order to explain hypnotic hallucination: the *imagination theory*, which is more clinical in nature; and the *holographic theory*, which is more transpersonal. Both are explained in more detail as follows:
A) Imagination Theory:
This theory defines hypnotic hallucination as simply figments of a person's imagination. An individual agrees to imagine something while under hypnosis, and it becomes enormously magnified in his or her mind's eye. Then later, upon experiencing the suggestion in the form of a post hypnotic suggestive experi-

ence, he or she experiences an imagination overlay.

For example, when people are told under hypnosis that upon awakening from hypnosis they will experience butterflies flying around their friend's head, they are simply imagining the butterflies with their eyes closed with such profound detail that the visual overlay is extraordinarily clear upon opening their eyes. The butterflies appear as a superimposed image over their friend's head. It can be so clear that often the part of consciousness that plays the role of the observer is laughing at the subject part of awareness (the part that is seeing the butterflies). All the while, the sum total of their experiences and perceptual awareness is giving them a natural balance for defining reality. In other words, individuals are very much aware that they are experiencing a hypnotic hallucination, so they enjoy the clarity of their imaginings.

In the chapter describing the laws of suggestion, we will find that a hypnotized individual must be motivated to experience a hallucination, in order for such a suggestion to properly manifest in an individual's experience. If an individual believes that acting silly is not going to be fun, he or she will deny the suggestion.

This is why most entertainment hypnosis shows are successful. Most of the volunteers have come forward with a willingness and motivation to acting silly. However, the individuals who have volunteered to participate in the show for the purpose of proving to the hypnotist that they can deny the suggestions are promptly told to leave the stage and return to their seats in the audience. This demonstrates how hypnotized individuals will never do anything against their morals, values, or better judgment. It also demonstrates how using imagination can be fun and harmless.

B) Holographic Theory:

Maybe the book, *The Holographic Universe*, explains the true nature of hypnotic hallucination when it tells of an experiment with a negative hallucination. A hypnotized subject is given the suggestion that someone in his environment is absent. The subject could then see *through* the person that was suggested away and accurately read an unspecified time on a clock being held behind the removed person's back. The suggested hypothesis was that the universe was holographic in nature, and the hypnotically absent person was not just a figment of imagination but, in effect, was dematerialized. Combining the power of the altered state with a person's imagination affects matter. We may actually be linked holographically to each other as part of a holographic universe. Wasn't it Albert Einstein who suggested that matter consists of particles of space and time, or that different forms of matter holds different spaces through differing vibratory rates? Are hypnotized people existing at a different vibratory rate which affects current time and space?

When we suggest that something is added or subtracted from a hypnotized subject's environment, it may actually be removed energetically from that person's world, internally and externally. If this is so, then maybe we *are* living in a holographic universe. If so, perhaps through hypnosis, we are materializing and dematerializing matter through thought. Perhaps we are actually able to access other planes of existence, such as memories and future projections, and these planes affect the physical/material realm here on earth. Maybe hypnosis affects the vibratory rates of different matter, and mind is the catalyst that makes this possible. Perhaps hypnosis, an altered state of consciousness, *is* the bridge for mind and matter, perhaps more so than we can currently comprehend.

In summary, various trance depths allow for different types of hypnotic phenomena to occur. Depending on the client's goal, hypnotherapists may choose to create deeper trance levels to ensure that the goal will be met. However, the deepest level of hypnosis, somnambulism—a sleep like state, would not be appropriate for regression, since the subject would have difficulty conversing with the hypnotherapist. As a general rule, medium deep levels of hypnosis are adequate for most therapeutic goals.

Chapter 14

Hypnotic Suggestion

Hypnotic suggestion leads people into various subjective realities which are often very clear and profoundly real within a client's imagination. Clients are much more likely to be led into these experiences when there is a good level of rapport and a therapeutic goal orientation. Some suggestions include ideas which lead an individual into a state of hypnosis (hypnotic induction), while some therapeutic suggestions emphasize futuristic creative conceptualization (post hypnotic suggestions). Some of these include imagery for healing the body, imagery for experiencing the superconscious or "spiritual" realities, imagery for spontaneously creating a solution to a problem, and more. Some suggestions are used strictly to create a reorientation effect for leading clients into remembering the past (hypnotic regression). The idea of *suggestion* will, therefore, overlap into several areas within the context of hypnotherapy throughout this text.

Suggestion takes place through people and their environments automatically every day. People cannot not communicate. In other words, a universal reality is that everyone on the planet is communicating something simply through their very existence. Therefore we are all giving messages to each other and our environment on a continual basis. During communication, a person's response to suggestions may be gauged by his or her body posture and facial expression. These reactions last only as long as a person concentrates on the topic being suggested. Suggestion is taking place regularly, which leads us to a broad definition of *waking suggestion*:

A stimulus which, through gaining one's attention, implants an idea in another person's mind, which is experienced within the subconscious imagery process as a reality, involuntarily and automatically, for as long as concentration is given to that particular subject matter.

Concentration is the only prerequisite for a person to experience hypnosis. Hypnosis takes the natural process of suggestion and amplifies it. Once hypnosis is achieved, everything is magnified in the person's subconscious imagery process, and through hypnosis, this magnification effect is suspended for a prolonged period of time. In hypnotic suggestion, the conscious mind is less active, so it is generally slower to interrupt a suggestion, as compared to the waking state. As a result, the subconscious mind's imagery experience is more vivid for a longer period of time, thus making the suggestion more of a reality. With this in mind, *hypnotic suggestion* may be defined as:

A stimulus which, while one is in a state of hypnosis, implants an idea in one's subconscious mind involuntarily and automatically, where it is amplified with vivification and remains a reality, until such point that it is suggested otherwise by the hypnotherapist or the subject.

Post-hypnotic suggestion is where a hypnotherapist gives a client a future oriented suggestion. This suggestion is either accepted or declined by the subject consciously or subconsciously. If it is accepted, the client generally experiences the suggestion as a vivid reality while under hypnosis. In other words, there is a sense of "living the future." Thereafter, upon awakening from hypnosis, at a specified moment in the future, and with the subject's awareness of a specified stimulus, the post hypnotic suggestion is triggered from the unconscious mind. This suggestion is often amnesiac, or lodged in the unconscious mind, and therefore is performed almost involuntarily and automatically. *Post-hypnotic Suggestion* may be defined as follows:

A stimulus which, while one is in a state of hypnosis, implants a futuristic idea in a person's subconscious mind, where it automatically becomes a reality with vivification. Upon awakening, and at a specific moment in time within the future, a stimulus triggers a response, or urge, to perform specific futuristic behaviors.

Generally, individuals will experience post hypnotic suggestions as an *urge* to perform a behavior, very similar to the urges of a typical self-programmed habit, such as smoking or eating. Normal habit urges are programmed into the unconscious mind from having life experiences. The urges that come from the unconscious mind that are programmed with hypnotic suggestion are experienced similarly.

For example, if we were to suggest to a smoker that he or she imagine having the mind and body of a nonsmoker in the future, and it is successfully imagined, it becomes at least as powerful as a memory of actually having lived the experience of being a nonsmoker. The difference is that this memory contains a future orientation. In essence, the subconscious mind actually receives the experience just as if an individual lived the experience in every day life.

In a sense, hypnosis provides us with new experiences without the need to actually go through these in the material world. Therefore, it assists us in quickly developing new resources that were previously unavailable. These new experiences give hypnotherapy clients more successful life experiences to draw upon. These quickly turn into daily resources leading to success and goal attainment.

The Five Laws of Suggestion

1) The law of familiarity
2) The law of truth and logic
3) The law of reverse effect
4) The law of dominant effect
5) The law of depth

1) <u>Familiarity:</u> The "path of least resistance" holds true for waking and hypnotic suggestion as well. Human nature is inclined to disregard a new idea in favor of one that is familiar. It is easier and less stressful. This is also true in hypnotherapy. Individuals are more likely to follow suggestions and post hypnotic suggestions that are familiar.

In other words, imagine if a hypnotherapist gave a female client two weight loss suggestions: one being that she will imagine fattening foods as bland Martian foods; and one being that fattening foods leave an oily residue in the mouth and throat. Within her everyday life, the woman is more familiar with the oily residue from fattening foods than she is with bland tasting Martian foods. As a result, she is more likely to accept the oily-residue suggestion, at least until we become educated that there is life on Mars and that Martians eat bland foods!

2) <u>Truth and Logic:</u> This law indicates that in order for an individual to accept a suggestion in the long term, it must be true for that person and make logical sense. If the suggestion is not true and logical, it will simply be considered a hallucination and thereby be disregarded during or shortly after the suggestion is given. It quickly loses its importance.

In other words, if a male smoking client is told that he will taste rotten fish upon putting a cigarette in his mouth, he may have brief experiences of disgust for possibly up to a 24 hour period. However, eventually homeostasis, or a state of natural balance, brings a person back to reality to understand that the suggestion was simply a temporary hypnotic hallucination. As a result, the client will probably begins smoking again, particularly if that was the only suggestion given to him. The suggestion was not based on true and logical ideas like black lungs, mucus, cancer, hospital visits, etc., of which are likely to last a lifetime.

3) <u>Reverse Effect:</u> The law of reverse effect indicates that imagination is stronger than will power. Often the general public holds the belief that a strong-willed person has a committed attitude that is more effective for change; once they are committed, they will follow through. However, without imagination, an in-

dividual cannot use the will to accomplish anything of significant value. In addition, the more difficult or distant the goal is, the more imagination required in order to achieve it. Many clients come into a hypnotherapy practice seeking more "willpower." The fact is that an individual must exercise his or her imagination to increase willpower. Our goal as imagination therapists then, is to teach individuals how to constructively use their imagination to benefit themselves. In a suggestive therapy format, we are teaching the client to imagine positive goal-oriented images involving the desired change, or current and past negative images involving the present problem. This form of imagination creates root-level motivation.

For some clients, imagination must be discussed and utilized with more detail, particularly if the goal for change is more monumental. Imagine that the goal is to walk across an oak plank of wood while remaining balanced. It requires very little effort to imagine doing so when the board is on the floor. It takes a little more effort to imagine walking across the plank when it is placed between two chairs. However, it will take a very intricate and detailed use of imagination to be able to walk across this plank when it is placed between two buildings. In fact, it may take the assistance of a hypnotherapist to amplify all of the details in order for success to occur. Once a hypnotherapist assists in a person's imagination, it becomes very natural for willpower to be there at the right time to create the highest amount of success.

4) <u>Dominant Effect:</u> The law of dominant effect claims that the strongest emotional desire will prevail. In other words, the suggestion with the strongest emotional desire attached to it will determine the behavioral outcome. This also includes the suggestions we give to ourselves from our own past programming, or our past experiences that are stored in the subconscious and unconscious areas of mind (see the Mind-Computer Model illustrated on the next page).

For an example, lets assume that a client has a goal of wearing a smaller swim suit at the beach this summer, but her biggest obstacle is the candy machine at work; so we give her the suggestion that as she walks by the candy machine at work, she will imagine herself this summer in a nice bathing suit and simply walk right past the candy machine, without partaking in the usual problematic eating behavior. Later, when she actually does become confronted with the candy machine at work, the strongest emotional desire will prevail. With all of the other laws of suggestion being constant, the question is, will she find the stronger drive for her behavior behind the post hypnotic suggestion of wearing the beautiful swimsuit on the beach, or behind the candy habit program of an immediate stress relief or reward at work? What will the client end up wanting? This makes the concept of *want* a very slippery word, one that is hard to determine.

This is why every hypnotherapist is destined to practice *strategic therapy*. This is where we take one week at a time with our clients, analyzing that which is and is not working for them from the last session—to determine the needs and interventions necessary for the current session. Fortunately, most hypnotherapy clients get results from the first session, provided effective therapy scripts are utilized, because they are highly motivated toward the changes they want.

Change generally stems from hypnotic suggestion, which results in a dominant effect. However, if the memory programs,

Mind-Computer Model

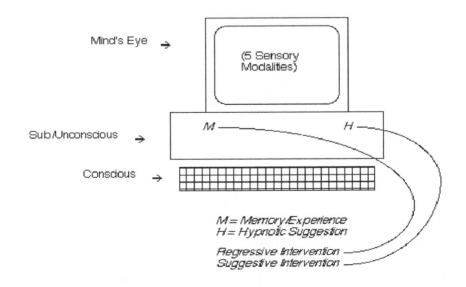

"M," prove to be more dominant than the hypnotic suggestions, "H," (in other words there is little to no change from the first session of suggestive therapy), then a hypnotherapist may consider using regressive hypnosis. Regression is commonly used to dismantle or re perceive the memory programs so that the hypnotic suggestions (which would then contain the strongest emotional desires) may prevail.

5) <u>Depth:</u> The deeper the trance level, generally the more likely suggestions will be accepted. This is because the conscious mind becomes less and less active as the client goes deeper into hypnosis. In the lighter levels of hypnosis, the conscious mind is more active and can intercept and change the suggestions more in accordance with the individual's conscious perceptions. The suggestions are also more readily heard and remembered. However, in the deeper levels of hypnosis, the client generally does not hear the suggestions given, at least on a conscious level; so the suggestions tend to meld with the unconscious mind and become unconscious ideas.

In the deeper level, the subject generally forgets what was told to them, which means the suggestions become amnesiac. Amnesiac suggestions are the most powerful, because they become urges or compulsions to think, feel, and behave certain ways. Students of hypnotherapy may think that deep levels of hypnosis are similar to mind control, when they actually are not. All of the other laws of suggestion must be satisfied, in order for there to be lasting results. However, when this one variable is utilized within this framework, the deeper trance levels will bring about a greater number of successes for goal attainment.

Personality and Inclination

Generally, whatever an individual is inclined to do in the waking state, or a normal state of consciousness, is what he or she will be willing to do while in hypnosis. It may be true that inhibitions are reduced, but not to an extreme. In other words, let's say our client has been a bank robber in the past, and he desires to rob another bank in the future, but just can't muster up the motivation to do so. He finds a psychotic hypnotist willing to give him the suggestions to imagine robbing the bank successfully. Because he is already inclined to do so, he is likely to follow through with it. This is not out of line with his character.

Contrarily, and hypothetically, if Sally, who has never even seriously imagined robbing a bank before, and was given this suggestion, she would simply laugh, deny the suggestion, wake up from hypnosis, or simply ignore the suggestion given forever. Sally was not inclined to rob a bank, so the hypnotic suggestion to do so was ineffective. I have never heard of either of these scenarios, thank goodness; however, they do illustrate the point behind the misconception of mind control. People will not do anything against their values, beliefs, or better judgment.

J. H. Conn[12] demonstrated through extensive experimentation that the idea of hypnotized subjects committing antisocial acts under hypnosis cannot be proven. Within the same stream of thought, a 1947 study[13] shows that self control is suppressed under hypnosis, but the flaw in this study becomes evident when they mention the use of military subjects. When given the suggestion to throw a bucket of acid on people from behind a wall of glass, the military subjects under hypnosis did so. However, it is my firm opinion, as well as the opinion of many other hypnosis researchers, that inclination is the determining factor. Such behaviors are also possible when the subjects are in the waking state. Military subjects are programmed to do what they are told. Conn also cites that the rapport and prestige of the hypnotist is also an important factor. In clinical hypnotherapy, if a client is *inclined* to change his or her behavior, he or she generally will do so and succeed.

Types of Suggestion

1) Negative   3) Direct
2) Positive   4) Indirect

1) <u>Negative suggestions</u> include negative words in them, such as "don't, won't, no, not, can't, shouldn't," and so on. They are given in such a manner as, "You won't experience..." or "you will not feel the urge to smoke." Because the subconscious mind takes every word literally and makes an image of them, these suggestions are 30% less effective. They are simply more confusing, since the subconscious mind does not process negatives as quickly and easily in hypnosis. The conscious mind, which is passive during hypnosis, is the expert at the process of elimination, or processing negatives, in order to create new meaning for the optimal behavior within the current circumstances.

In the waking state, there are two steps: the subconscious mind first shows imagery of what not to do; then it shows imagery geared toward that which we are to do instead. In hypnosis, the second stage does not take place as easily. The subconscious mind imagines what not to do, and unfortunately, that is what it has been frequently doing before a client enters into hypnotherapy for a habitual problem. For these reasons, unless the client states their motivations for change with negative semantics, these should not be utilized in suggestive scripts.

2) <u>Positive suggestions</u> are a combination of semantics that are void of negative words, (i.e.., "You will experience...") and they contain future outcomes. The client of hypnosis is told what he or she is to experience at that moment, or at sometime in the future (post hypnotic). According to research, positive suggestions are 30% more effective than negative suggestions. When selecting suggestive therapy scripts and induction scripts, the wise hypnotherapist would best choose the scripts that contain a majority of positive, outcome-based suggestions.

3) <u>Direct suggestions</u> are simply more direct in nature, (i.e.. "Close your eyes"). These suggestions can be used in both clinical and entertainment settings. Clinical Hypnotherapists tend to use these to direct their client toward that which they want the client to do, (e.g. "You will stop overeating in the evenings at home"). Stage hypnotists tend to use these suggestions as part of their authoritarian approach, for the entertainment value during their

shows, (e.g. "Sleep!" or "When I snap my fingers you'll____").

4) Indirect suggestions are given during normal conversation, most often during the pre-session or post-session interviews. Milton Erickson was the master of indirect suggestion, and many language patterns loaded with subtle suggestions were observed and decoded by John Grinder and Richard Bandler, the creators of Neurolinguistic Programming. These patterns contain presuppositions which can be used to create new meanings for clients, (i.e. "When *now* did you want to make this change"). The client will often respond with, "Well, I think right *now*." They are unconscious of the word "now" stated in the question as the answer. This response in the pre-session interview often leads to less resistance and a greater chance for success. Story telling metaphors or inductions are also generally loaded with indirect suggestions for change.

The real therapeutic value in suggestion and post hypnotic suggestion is that people are able to replace old habits with new ones. As long as the new habits are as much or more satisfying than the old ones, they could last indefinitely. Over a period of time, post hypnotic suggestions become a conditioned response. Clients simply experience the habit of having a different life style, and in most cases it results in permanent change.

The laws of suggestion dictate therapeutic outcomes. There is no magic, when it comes to people accepting suggestions, even though clients often are surprised at the changes that take place when they did not have to consciously work at them. If suggestions were accepted automatically and involuntarily, they would be referred to as commands. Nonetheless, hypnotherapy is known as a back door approach, since it involves internal changes that require little effort beyond the therapy sessions, unlike counseling or psychotherapy. Although these methods have unique merits under certain circumstances, it is said that when comparing the two, one session of hypnotherapy is worth 10 sessions of counseling or psychotherapy. In many cases, hypnotherapy tends to be quicker and more effective.

Chapter 15

Self-Hypnosis and Hypnomeditation

The pioneer of self-hypnosis was Emil Coue (1857-1926). His favorite auto suggestion, or self-hypnosis suggestion, was, "Everyday, in every way, I am getting better and better." Self-Hypnosis, is the process by which an individual puts himself or herself under hypnosis. Compared to hetero-hypnosis, where a hypnotherapist puts us under hypnosis, obtaining trance is less effective, unless we are well practiced with self-hypnosis skills. It is not as easy for us to put ourselves under hypnosis, because it requires that we play more than one role, the therapist, the client, and the observer. In hetero-hypnosis, it is easier for us to enter a state of hypnosis, because all we have to do is imagine what is being described to us. The task of formulating suggestions is done by somebody else, so it is easier for us to simply have the experience that someone else provides.

In the book, *Hypnosis: Research Developments and Perspectives*, it is theorized by E. Fromm that the ego is split into 3 parts. These are listed below.

1. Speaker- formulates suggestions
2. Listener- experiences the suggestions
3. Observer- examines the effect of the suggestions
   If we were to look at the illustration below, we would notice

the categorization of the three main parts of the ego with different but similar labels. I refer to these as the three primary parts of consciousness, or "trifold consciousness." This includes: the operator, (which suggests the ideas); the subject, (which receives the ideas and experiences them); and the observer, (the part of consciousness that oversees the process). These functions are in operation during a normal state of consciousness, as well as in self-hypnosis. However, within a hypnotherapy session, the operator role is performed by the hypnotherapist, who is formulating the suggestions with and for the client..

Tri-Fold Consciousnes¦

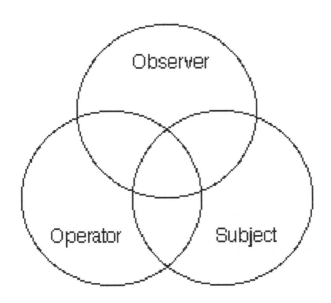

During hetero-hypnosis, when somebody else is giving the suggestions, our subconscious mind receives them in the form of imagery and our conscious mind, the observer, observes and makes decisions about the effectiveness of the process. This is why it is said that we cannot completely detach the ego, or the conscious mind, while in hypnosis. The ego refers to the observer. The ego releases control but is still active to some degree, although less active as the trance level deepens.

It has been said that *all hypnosis is self-hypnosis*, because it occurs inside of an individual and it is not an external event. Even in hetero-hypnosis, a hypnotherapist suggests ideas for relaxation and imagination, but the client has the final say, figuratively speaking, as to how much he or she wants to internalize and experience those suggestions. We must participate in agreeing to imagine the suggestions, or in other words, hypnotize ourselves with the ideas that are suggested.

Important Uses of Self-Hypnosis:

1. Pain management- Because some individuals will need regular pain relief, it is often best for them to learn self-hypnosis with pain management tools. The benefit to this is that they can apply these tools to themselves, when needed (while experiencing discomfort), at any time in the future. In addition, it keeps the client conditioned to hypnosis, so that it remains effective for relief.

2. Conditioning between hypnotherapy sessions- Many professional hypnotherapists believe that taping suggestive therapy sessions, for the client to listen to between appointments, increases results. In general, self-hypnosis tapes and C.D.s are theorized to improve depth levels, and also create a greater conditioned response to therapeutic suggestions. In private practice, it is best to start taping from the beginning of the induction, through the therapy suggestions, and all the way to the end of the awakening procedures, stopping the tape there.

3. Putting ourselves to sleep- Many individuals have taken self-hypnosis courses for the purpose of releasing daily stresses, and reducing the problems associated with falling asleep. It is known to be highly effective to use a mixed induction on ourselves, particularly emphasizing progressive relaxation while lying in bed. Often, before the end of the induction, the individual has fallen asleep.

4. Improve meditation- Entering meditation using the self-hypnosis techniques outlined in this chapter is very beneficial for increasing the depth of the meditative state. We would start with self-hypnosis, reach a sufficient depth, and then proceed into the meditative experiences from there. This is particularly useful for transcendental meditation.

5. Improve performance- Using self-hypnosis before performances (such as public speaking, medical procedures, sports, business meetings, and more), increases concentration levels, relaxation, mental clarity, attitude, and productivity. One of the most valuable techniques to teach athletes involves using self-hypnosis with imagery for imagining the most successful movements (strokes, swings, runs, etc.) immediately before the sports event begins.

6. Counteract stress- Research shows that doing one or two self-hypnosis inductions on ourselves each day boosts the immune system and reduces the stress response—which is responsible for cardiovascular problems, and more. Self-hypnosis proves to be very beneficial for health and wellness with just 10 minute sessions.

Common Difficulties with Self-Hypnosis:

1. Dual function- Performing the function of both formulating suggestions and receiving or imagining them tends to lighten the trance level. It often can turn into self talk, if the practitioner of self-hypnosis is not careful to keep the rules for success in mind, particularly the one which advises us to condense the suggestions (more on this below).

2. Falling asleep- Sometimes, a practitioner of self-hypnosis will lose self talk in the deeper trance level and fall asleep. This is because of the fact that people tend to give themselves suggestions to relax and "sleep" just before falling asleep at bed time. If we tend to fall asleep trying self-hypnosis, one way to help ourselves stay in the state between awake and asleep is to say to ourselves,

"I will go as deep as possible and remain aware of everything." This can be said before or during the induction.

Rules for Successful Self-Hypnosis Sessions:

a) <u>Use a depth test-</u> Sometimes we can use a sign of hypnosis to recognize when we are under hypnosis. One of the signs I like to use for myself is the arms going numb. Another indicator is when the arm rises up from the lap using a balloon imagination test.

b) <u>Sit in an upright position-</u> Sitting in an upright position on the floor or against a wall, as opposed to soft, comfortable furniture, reduces the common problem of falling asleep.

c) <u>Condense all suggestions-</u> It is best to only formulate one to three sentences to use as suggestions for self-hypnosis. This helps avoid lightening the trance from excessive self-talk.

d) <u>Future orientation-</u> Make sure that all suggestions are future oriented. This will facilitate a positive attitude toward that which we want to occur, rather than that which we are trying to avoid. Suggestions about past problems can cause us excessive stress and reduce chances for a successful future.

e) <u>Make suggestions true and logical-</u> As with the laws of suggestion, it is important to create suggestions to be true for our life-style. If the suggestions are logical, they will last much longer, or perhaps indefinitely.

f) <u>Utilize a good mixed induction-</u> As always, the mixed method (imagery and progressive relaxation) is going to be the most successful for a broad range of personalities.

Five Types of Auto Suggestion

1) <u>Verbal / Aloud-</u> This type of suggestion is used while we are under hypnosis. At that time, we begin to repeat the suggestion aloud in a speaking or whispering voice.

2) <u>Verbal / Internal-</u> This type of suggestion is also given while in trance as we mentally rehearse the words to ourselves.

3) <u>Imagery-</u> Imagery should be future oriented and include the three main sensory modalities of visual, auditory, and kinesthetic, if possible. The student of self-hypnosis either imagines: 1) an event that represents the process it will take to become successful; and / or 2) the end result of having already achieved success. It can be most beneficial to select the image before undergoing trance, but also the imagery which often spontaneously surfaces during trance tends to be very beneficial.

4) <u>Pre Hypnotic-</u> This tool involves rehearsing the suggestions to ourselves before inducing hypnosis. This method is like using an affirmation, and then there is an awareness automatically that the trance is done for the purpose of such affirmation.

5) <u>Taped-</u> Many individuals like to tape their induction and a lengthy script of suggestions, followed up with the normal awakening procedures. In essence, we are giving ourselves a full hypnosis session. However, an important factor for success is that we must enjoy the sound of our own voice on tape. Many of us do not, because of the different sound quality we hear when our voices are not vibrating the bones within our heads, such as the case when speaking.

Self-Hypnosis and Hypnomeditation Procedures

The primary purpose of the following exercise is to relax the mind and body to a level as close to the sleep state as possible without losing consciousness. The secondary purpose, which is to reach a deeper state likened to meditation, is to reduce or eliminate the activity of the conscious mind and create an effect by which we experience dissociating from our environment and ascending into a different, higher reality. To begin with, by relaxing the body and pacifying the conscious mind, and then clearing ourselves of our stresses, we may reach deep levels of the altered state. This deeper level is required for achieving transcendental meditation. If the practitioner desires, he or she may perform the second step in the transpersonal self-hypnosis procedures labeled, "transcendental meditation segment."

Learning Self-Hypnosis:

Learning self-hypnosis is rather easy for students of hypnotherapy, because they have already learned to apply inductions and suggestions on others. It is easier to apply our education on ourselves, than if we were learning about hypnosis for the first time.

Self-Hypnosis Procedures

1) Position- Sit in a lightly padded chair or against the wall. Support your back so that it is in a straight position you can maintain for a period of time. Uncross your legs (reducing cramping), separate your hands (reducing distraction), and close your eyes.

2) Imagery- Choose a safe place in nature where you are able to create a relaxing reality, project to the future, or go to a place where you have been before and have felt very relaxed. Often, the best memory imagery is a place where you have meditated before. Use the imagination to sharpen visual, auditory, and kinesthetic sensory modalities.

3) Progressive Relaxation- Imagine a wave of sunlight representing goodness, or the light of the creator, flowing from head to toe. As it moves through each muscle group, relax that area to its fullest. Concentrate on deep, slow rhythmic breathing. Move

the stress out with each exhale.

4) Deepening- Repeat relaxing words to yourself ("relax", "deeper" etc....) and include the phrase, "I'll go as deep as possible without entering sleep." Then, any deepening technique from the related chapter on such will be beneficial.

5) Clearing- Allow your awareness to notice anything within yourself (mentally or physically) that may be of a stressful or negative nature (i.e.. anger, resistance, guilt, un-forgiveness, etc.) and release it into the source of the light. Now, the practitioner of self-hypnosis may proceed to step six below, and add twenty to sixty minutes to the allotted time, or go to step 8 and awaken.

Transcendental Meditation Segment:

6) Transcendence- After fully clearing your mind and body, put a protective bubble of white light around your body and allow your consciousness to transcend into the light for a visual, auditory, or kinesthetic awareness for guidance—seeing, hearing, or feeling a bright loving guide, or guides. Anything cartoon-like or negative, send away to the light and move closer to the light until you have qualified a stable apparition of a loving being or angelic guide.

7) Communion- You may bring a question or simply listen for those things that are most important for you to telepathically hear or understand at this time in your life. If your mind is relaxed enough, you will lose the logical mind and be clear enough to receive divine messages or impressions.

8) Awakening- Ask to remember all the important things you've experienced, and move your consciousness back into your body slowly, in order to facilitate remembering. When you are back and aware of the present, say to yourself, "wide awake and feeling good." You may even count yourself back from "3 to 1." When reaching "1," you may awaken. Other Awakening procedures are listed below.

Remember, your guides are always there to assist you with anything you need and will generally tell you what you need to know or understand about your purpose within the time zone from which you are transcending. There may be occasions where you will already know the answer you are seeking, or times you may feel the question is inconsequential as compared to the experience you are having in the meditation, particularly if you are reaching the akashic records—(the place of all knowledge). Relax, and enjoy, remembering to return. A return trip is easier the more you practice self-hypnosis.

Self-Hypnosis Awakening Procedures

Most students of self-hypnosis will be in trance for five to fifteen minutes, while the student of hypnomeditation may be in hypnosis and transcendental meditative dimensions for up to two hours. Once an individual has been under hypnosis for an adequate amount of time, the following awakening procedures may be used.

1) <u>Visualize face of clock-</u> Before we go into trance, we may mentally set a time to awaken. While under hypnosis, the face of the clock enters into our mind automatically when it is the right time, almost as if the subconscious contains its own internal alarm clock. While we have been under hypnosis for an adequate period of time, we can visualize the face of a clock and then open our eyes or perform the count-back awakening procedures listed previously.

2) <u>Length of time-</u> Before we go into trance, we plot out the length of time desired. After inducing trance, we sense that the predetermined length of time has expired and we either simply open our eyes, or perform a count-back procedure.

In general, practitioners of self-hypnosis are more successful if they are dedicated to the study of hypnosis and practice
self-hypnosis regularly. The best way to condition the self to self-
hypnosis more rapidly is for the student of hypnosis to first have
a hypnotherapist put him or her into a deep level of hypnosis.
Once this is accomplished, we obtain a deeper level than what we
could have obtain by ourselves, developing a pathway into the
unconscious mind and thereby making it easier to use the same
pathway more successfully in the future. In addition, the likelihood of falling asleep is decreased, when another person is present
assisting the exercise.

Some research shows that individuals reach their goals more
easily with self-hypnosis, as compared to hetero-hypnosis, while
other research indicates that a facilitator is more effective. It is my
opinion that it depends on the personality type. We may want to
ask ourselves, "Am I generally self-motivated, or would I do better
confronting this problem with somebody else's direct assistance?"
It may be possible for students of self-hypnosis to reach therapeutic
goals on their own, provided they are experienced practitioners
of the art, and the goals are not too monumental.

For further education in self-hypnosis, I advise readers to
obtain the book, *Self-Hypnosis: Creating Your Own Destiny*, by Henry
Bolduc, which is listed on the publisher page in the afterward of
this book. It offers a well-rounded, transpersonal approach, with
several enlightening concepts that are based in the work of Edgar
Cayce. Several hypnotherapists have been known to use Henry
Bolduc's book to teach courses in self-hypnosis at community colleges, institutions, and more.

The benefits of self-hypnosis are numerous. For we hypnotherapists, self-hypnosis is an ideal method for clearing ourselves
of issues that may stand in the way of rapport and greater success
with our clients. On a broader level, most people in our stressful,
quick-paced society can obtain multiple benefits from learning
and practicing self-hypnosis on a regular basis.

Chapter 16

Client Interview

There are three forms that new clients receive upon entering my office. The first is a "Confidential Interview" form, which requests name, address, some medical and psychological information describing what kind of therapy or treatment modalities were used in the past, and why the client seeks hypnotherapy treatment. The second is a "Policies" form, which is a contract describing what the client is responsible for (fees, treatment programs, etc.) and may expect as a result of utilizing hypnotherapy. The third form is titled, "What is hypnotherapy?," which has been outlined in a previous chapter. If clients answer these questions for themselves beforehand in the waiting room, then when they enter into the treatment room, their concerns may have already been alleviated. This way, the client and I spend less time discussing what hypnosis is and is not (misconceptions, etc.) and focus more time on the specific issue he or she wants to address.

In some form, the aforementioned documents are generally included in the training manual of the hypnotherapy training institution that a student of hypnotherapy is attending. Another form, used for interviewing the client, is filled out by the practitioner by their eliciting information directly from the client during an interview. This is called the "Client Interview" form and is the foundation for this chapter.

The ability to interview a client, and thereby gain rapport, is probably the single most important factor for maximizing success. Although it takes time for the new hypnotherapist to develop good interview skills, it is worth performing a dozen or so of these procedures, in order to gain proficiency. This is what primarily increases a hypnotherapist's success rate above and beyond the success achieved from simply reading induction and therapy scripts. Although the interview form taught in this chapter, when adequately completed, automatically gains rapport, there is no replacement for the proficiency gained from interviewing a wide variety of clients over a period of time.

Rapport

Milton Erickson said that the most important factor for achieving a successful induction is establishing rapport. Rapport is described as experiencing a feeling of being understood. When two people are in rapport, there is a dance that takes place, which can be observed as similarities in body posture, vocal tones, and behavior patterns. This process, used by many NLP Practitioners, hypnotherapists, and sales managers in various corporations, is referred to as "matching and mirroring." It is done automatically and unconsciously with those individuals who are in rapport (e.g. the client reclines back in his or her chair with hands behind the head, and therefore so does the therapist, as if looking at himself or herself in the mirror).

Gaining rapport with clients can be learned through the study of neurolinguistic programming (NLP), which emphasizes conscious matching and mirroring techniques. Although these tools may be helpful, the best way to establish rapport, rather, is to demonstrate a genuine interest in the client's problems and goals. This is generally done through a mixture of exercising compassion, asking pertinent questions that encompass the client's problem, and using good listening skills. The foundation to executing these is the client interview form, such as the one illustrated later in this chapter. Once rapport is established, matching and mirroring are automatic, and miraculous changes often result.

Four steps for gaining rapport

1) Self Clearing- This self-hypnosis exercise should be done before each day, so that hypnotherapists may be clear of their own personal problems before addressing those of their clients. By referring to the chapter on self-hypnosis, we will notice the step whereby we clear any negative thought or feeling by imagining where in the mind or body we are storing these. We release them into the light at the beginning of the self-hypnosis exercise. A more indirect way to clear ourselves may involve the spiritual practice of inviting the higher forces into our sessions before seeing our first client.

2) Small Talk- This can be accomplished by talking about the weather, something in the office—like a picture of our family, or some other ordinary topic of conversation. Small talk should last about one to five minutes. If it goes much beyond that, there may be the impression given by either party that a most important topic is being avoided for some reason. Generally, small talk relaxes both practitioner and client. It socially warms up the client and avoids prematurely jumping into problem-oriented topics before the client is at ease enough to discuss them.

3) Investigator Role- The next step is to play the role of investigator. This is accomplished by our following a series of questions that brings out a brief history of the problem through the present moment, and then into the kind of future we desire. At that point, the present circumstances are asked about in detail (i.e. when, where, and specifically how the problem takes place). While playing this role, the client is doing 99% of the sharing and the therapist is asking very direct questions that will lead toward clarity. Under the client centered approach, the therapist is not leading the client by asking presumptive questions, or trying to diagnose the problem for the client. The therapist is not suggesting anything, in any way. The answers to the client's problems are inherent in the asking of pertinent questions that are derived from the client interview form.

4) Co-creator Role- This role involves Co-creating ideas with the client, during the interview, that the client deems important for him or her to be able make the desired changes. Once a

general picture of the problem is drawn out of the client, (triggers, patterns, and goals) we begin to formulate suggestions together with the client. If we are at a loss in developing counter suggestions (reframing triggers and patterns), we can simply ask, "What is it that your subconscious mind needs to hear concerning this (trigger/pattern)?" and then write these concepts down for using them as suggestions when the client is under trance. It is imperative that we remember that clients have all of the answers within themselves, in order to solve their problems. It is simply our job as a facilitator to help the client discover these during the interview, or within the scope of a hypnotic regression—if necessary as a secondary procedure.

The Co-creator role is perhaps the most important step in the interview process for increasing success rates of suggestive therapy scripts. This is where the concept comes into play that a hypnotherapist's greatest asset is *creativity*. As reperceptual therapists, we recreate old realities into new realizations that are beneficial for the client to comprehend consciously during the interview. Thereafter, during the trance, the full power of that which has been discovered in the interview can be suggested to the subconscious mind where it is thereby realized more quickly in the process of change.

Habit Analysis and Intervention

The process of habit analysis and intervention is the primary goal of the client interview. Since all problems contain patterns, or repetitive behaviors, the client interview in this book can be used for virtually any therapeutic goal. It is designed so that as we ask pertinent questions about the problems and goals, the client will automatically discover patterns, or habitual problematic behaviors.

Habit patterns underlie almost every behavior, particularly for adults since their unconscious minds have a lot more information stored in them than youth do. The unconscious mind stores habitual behaviors so that the conscious mind can focus on learning new experiences. The more experiences that are stored in the limitless storehouse of the unconscious mind, the more versatile abilities we have. Most unconscious behaviors are forgotten, or are unavailable to the conscious mind, but yet exist in a powerfully automatic way. We are a sum total of all of all of our experiences, all of which are stored in the unconscious mind as memories.

We may discuss the unconscious programming of our client by focusing on pertinent memories thereby pinpointing the problem and transforming it more rapidly. Because of the effectiveness of the associative-motivational method that I designed (see following illustration), sometimes changes take place before hypnosis and suggestions are used. However, most of the time, hypnotic suggestion is the key ingredient for transforming unconscious mental processes and shifting compulsions and urges into more productive directions. The client interview both establishes a profound level of rapport and uniquely individualizes the session.

The Associative-Motivational Method

As we focus on the illustration that follows, we will notice that there is space on the client interview form for documenting two sessions, the first and the second. If there are more than two sessions given to a client, the "Session II" section of the form may be used for subsequent interviews.

Association- *A thought, idea, or behavior (stimulus) which automatically triggers another thought, idea, or behavior (response).*

Motivation- *A positive movement mentally and physically toward a pleasurable outcome, or a negative movement mentally and physically away from a unpleasant outcome.*

Secondary Gain- *A major benefit derived consciously or unconsciously from maintaining a problematic condition, so much so that it is difficult or impossible to relinquish the stated problem.*

In the first session, so that rapport is developed more effectively, using chronology, it is advisable to list early associations first, current day associations next, and then motivations last. The client's *early associations, current associations,* and *secondary gains* should be listed on the left side of the form first, and then his or her *positive motivations* and *negative motivations* would be listed on the right side of the page.

Client Interview Form

Session I:

Associations   **Motivations: +/-**
(Counter Suggestions)

Early:

Current:

Secondary Gains:

Session II:

New Associations   **Effective Changes**

(end of form)

Early Associations:
        These are elicited from the client by asking the question, "What are your earliest memories related to the problem?" For weight loss, it might be that parents told their children (your clients) to clean their plates. For a smoking client, it might be that a sibling, who the client looked up to, offered them cigarettes. For a pain management client, it might be that a car accident was the first time back problems began. Patterns begin in various ways.

Current Associations:
        These are elicited from the client by asking the question, "What things in the current day are associated with the problem?" For weight loss, it might be that the client only eats at night. For a smoking client, he or she may only smoke during social occasions. For the pain management client, he or she may experience more pain while traveling in an automobile on long trips. Current day associations are numerous, in the cases of common habits, such as smoking and weight, and make up a long list on the left side of the form.

Secondary Gains:
        These are elicited from the client by asking the question, "What major benefit is there, if any, to maintaining this problem?" For the weight loss client, it might be that being over weight provides the benefit of protection. This could be protection from the opposite sex, criminals, and more. For the smoking client, it might be that he or she really doesn't want to live a long life. For the pain client, it could be that the pain frequently allows for days off from work. This area may or may not exist for clients, as most of them will answer "no" to the question. In some cases, the realization that these exist is a surprise. In these cases, it is essential to a client's success to discuss and formulate a key counter suggestion, removing any significant counter motivation to change. This leads us to counter-suggestions...

Counter-Suggestions:
        On the left hand side of the page, on the client interview form, we should leave room for counter suggestions to be listed

under each association. Each association is underlined and reframing is exercised. In the book *Reframing*, Richard Bandler and John Grinder indicate that every problematic behavior has a positive intention. Once that positive intention is discovered, new healthier behaviors of equal or superior value can replace the old ones.

In other words, the positive intentions of old-problematic behaviors may be rechanneled through more positive, happier and healthier behaviors. It is as if there is an unconscious part of ourselves, an urge, that needs to be satisfied through some sort of behavior, which is particularly true for habits. Since almost every problem is habitual, this concept can be utilized successfully for almost every hypnotherapeutic goal.

For a smoking client that uses cigarettes for creating and taking work breaks, we may ask them how they will still satisfy the need to take work breaks as a nonsmoker. For a weight client who uses food to alleviate boredom, we may ask what other activities can be suggested that are healthy and alleviate boredom, and so on. We increase our success rate by going through a list of options for replacement habits. Although it takes the new hypnotherapist time to discuss these in an educated way, the client is even further in the dark, not fully consciously aware of habit triggers, etc., so we can be assured that even the most basic questions are thought provoking enough when we are starting out.

Freud theorized that there is a force seeking an outlet; and when that outlet is blocked, the force seeks another outlet. This is why he was an advocate of what he referred to as symptom treatment and advised against symptom removal. In fact, he said that symptom removal was counterproductive or dangerous to many clients who used hypnosis in his day, because the new outlet, or habit, which replaced the old one, when it was suggested away by hypnosis, may be worse than the original problem (e.g. a person stops smoking and starts drinking alcohol excessively). However, this is less likely to be the case for the client who comes to see a hypnotherapist in our current era. Most hypnotherapy clients are more functional, having far less neurosis than those who Freud saw as clients years ago for psychoanalysis. Nonetheless, as a general rule, reframing associations into counter-suggestions allows for symptom treatment, not symptom removal, and symptom treatment is most effective.

Secondary gains need to be looked at closely, and the question should be posed to the client, "How can you accomplish this goal differently?" In the case of the weight loss client, let's assume that the client responded that there was a major benefit for maintaining the problem and that it was because she didn't want to be asked out for a date anymore; she gave up on intimate relationships after her last break up. She was hurt, so she lost the desire to look thin and attractive. The purpose for having the extra weight was protection, so we ask her the counter-suggestion elicitation question above, and she responds, "I guess that I can just tell men that I'm not interested when I'm thin, if I don't want to get romantically involved." This answers how she can get the same benefit differently; she decided to verbally say "no," instead of physically saying "no" with her body, so this statement is written below the secondary gain as a counter suggestion.

Motivations:

These are elicited from clients by asking, "For what reasons are you making this change?" The key word for elicitation is "reasons," because the client has been thinking about many of these before calling a hypnotherapist's office for an appointment. The client will list several reasons. For weight loss clients, they usually involve health and self image. For other interventions, we will elicit a variety of motivations that are very unique to that person. Eliciting motivations is generally the last step of the interview process, before inducing hypnosis.

Let's look at a typical example of a weight loss interview that is different from the one just mentioned above. We will assume a fictitious name for a male client who's name is "John."

Weight Loss Interview Example-John:

Reframing a weight loss client's early association of "clean your plate" may be done by asking the client, "What is it that you would like me to tell your subconscious mind about cleaning your plate?" In this case, let's say that our client, John, said, "Tell me that I don't need to eat out of guilt anymore. Also tell me that I can make a small annual donation to starving children. You know, I would just like to push the food away from me when I'm full, so that I don't overeat anymore." (See the weight loss interview illustration that follows.)

Also, we can use positive intention reframing and ask, "What is it that you are getting from eating all of the food on your plate?" "I guess I feel like I'm doing the right thing" might be the client's answer. It could be noted to the client that feeling like doing the right thing for themselves and others may be accomplished by taking less food, leaving food on their plate now, or saving the food for later. Hopefully the client will agree and then those are the suggestions used as the counter-suggestions.

Let's say that John told us that he feels that eating food at night is a reward for a hard day at work, then we can ask, "What other rewards at night can you provide yourself that make you feel good?" The client may say, "I give myself negative self-talk, I guess I just need to hear more positive messages from my subconscious that I did my best and I deserve to relax." We can also ask the client what else he needs to hear, and he might say, "Tell me the kitchen is off limits, I just seem to wander into it and eat without thinking about it." He might also say, "I need to be able to resist the refrigerator...I wish I could just imagine a big red X on the refrigerator at night." In this case, we formulate these suggestions close to verbatim, using as many of the client's own words as possible, as in the following illustration.

For example, in the event that there are secondary gains, let's assume that John said "yes" that there was a major benefit for maintaining the problem and that it was because he wanted to be heavy enough to win in the event of a physical challenge or assault. The weight's purpose is protection, so we ask him about a counter suggestion, and he says, "I guess that I can lose weight and exercise so that I am even more strong and capable." This answers how he can maintain the same benefit and be healthy, so this statement is written below the secondary gain as a counter suggestion.

Next we list John's motivations as he states them word for word verbatim. They are either negative or positive motivations. Motivations are based in the pain pleasure principle, whereby we move away from pain and toward pleasure. Negative motivations represent pain, and positive motivations represent pleasure. As John tries to move away from the unpleasant conditions of being overweight, we mark those motivations with an "N." As he states positive concepts that he will enjoy about being thin in the future, we list these with a "P."

Note John's interview form #1, weight loss session #1, which follows.

John's Interview Form #1

Weight Loss Session I:

Associations

(Early)
Clean Your Plate (Guilt)
"You're free from eating for reasons of guilt"
"Making your annual donation to the hungry"
"You will be doing the right thing for yourself and others by pushing food away when full"

stairs."
(Current)
talk."
Negative Self-talk
"You'll tell yourself that you did your best, that's good enough, and you deserve to relax"

Rewards at night
"You'll reward yourself at night with other things than food"
"You'll avoid eating food at night, putting it out of you mind, forgetting about it"

Unconsciously wanders into kitchen at night
"The kitchen will be off limits at night when you consistently imagine a red 'X' on the refrigerator."

(Secondary Gains)
Protection from danger
"You can lose weight and therefore become even more strong and capable."

Motivations: +/-

P-*"want to live longer."*
N-*"tired of feeling tired."*
N-*"joints hurt."*
P-*"want to enjoy life again."*
P- *"have a healthier heart."*
P-*"feel like exercising more."*
P- *"have more energy for*

N- *"eliminate negative self*

Linking Suggestions

Once the form for session one is complete, the next step is to put John under hypnosis and read to him all of the counter suggestions and his motivations. One of the best ways a hypnotherapist can do this is by tying these statements together with what I refer to as "because statements" and conjunctions, such as:

"Because of (a counter-suggestion), you will (a motivation)." This has been done below from John's session #1 interview form:

1A. *"Because you'll avoid eating for reasons of guilt—you will live longer."*
1B. *"Because you're making your annual donation to the hungry, you'll stop eating all the food on your plate and you will never feel tired again"*
1C. *"Because you will be doing the right thing for yourself by pushing food away, your joints will stop hurting."*
1D. *"Because you'll reward yourself at night with other things than food, you'll begin to enjoy life again."*
1E. *"Because you'll avoid eating food at night, putting it out of you mind, forgetting about it, you will have a healthier heart."*
1F. *"Because you'll imagine a red "X" on the refrigerator at night, you'll know that the kitchen will be off limits and you will become thinner and feel like exercising more."*
1G. *"Because you're thin, you will be stronger and more capable and you will eliminate all negative self-talk from entering into your mind.*

Note that if there are more or less counter suggestions than motivations, the best thing to do is repeat one of the motivations or counter suggestions in the list. Another alternative, is to make up an obvious motivations, such as "health."

Thereafter, if we choose *linking,* it is important to ad-lib. Keep in mind that linking is not mandatory for obtaining results; we could simply read off the counter suggestions and motivations while the client is in trance and get good results. As long as the client's own words are utilized in the statements, they will most likely be effective. This is a key component to the client interview process, because the client's own words are internal representations of subconscious associations.

The purpose of session one is to create new changes, while the purpose of session two is to create the perception that the changes that have taken place are not temporary (i.e.. smoking clients that still believe they are smokers who are temporarily abstaining from cigarettes, when ideally it is best for their perceptual reality to become that of a "nonsmoker" who has mastered the change permanently).

Session II:

In subsequent sessions, the lower portion of the client interview form can be utilized. Essentially the client is going to be listing the changes that have taken place over the past few days or a week. Then, they will list any new associations that have surfaced since the last session, or the old associations that have not yet been changed. These are then reframed as counter-suggestions, the effective changes are listed and then linking may take place, as in John's case.

At some point shortly after the beginning of the second session, we may ask John, "Well, how did everything go after your first session?" Let's assume John says, "Good, I really noticed a desire to stay away from the kitchen. I remember this big red 'X' appeared on the refrigerator. Wow, the imagination is really powerful, isn't it? Also, I started already feeling like I was losing some weight. I feel lighter and like I already have more energy, but I was wondering if you could give me a suggestion that would help me stop snacking. I think that if I could stop snacking during the day, I would do even better. Maybe I do it out of boredom..."

Now at this point, we want to reframe the snacking into a counter-suggestion. We may also look back at the lists from Session-one and ask, "Well John, it sounds good, but I was also wondering about some other associations, like, how is the self-talk coming?" John may answer, "real positive." We may also ask, "How do you feel about protection and weight?" Let's say that John responded to this as, "I'm feeling stronger and healthier now that I'm losing weight." Notice how these are listed as in the following interview form for session two.

John's Interview Form #2

Session II:

New Associations	**Effective Changes**
Daytime snacking	*Desire to stay away from refrigerator*
Alleviate boredom with	*Positive self talk*
interesting thoughts/activities	*Seeing a big red 'X' on the refrigerator*
	Feel lighter, more energy

Although we could suggest to John the counter suggestions under "New Associations" and the list of "Effective Changes" at some point after the hypnotic induction, and still obtain results, linking suggestions is a nice tool. If we choose linking suggestions in session-two, it involves the same process as in session-one, except a few additional techniques. In John's case, we will link the counter suggestions from the new association list to the motivations in the motivation list derived from session-one. This sustains motivation through session-two and beyond. In this example, we do this again with "because-statements":

2A. "Because you are alleviating snacking with interesting thoughts and healthier activities, you will notice that you are reaching your goals of (read off all motivations listed in motivations list from session-one)."

2B. "Because you are a thinner person, you're now realizing many satisfying changes have taken place permanently (read off all changes in the effective changes list from session-two)."

If we ever start wondering what the next step is in the interview process, we can always do what Erickson recommended, "Trust the Unconscious (of our client)." This means that every person knows the answers to his or her problem, at least unconsciously. Clients spent years getting to know themselves, and therefore they know themselves better than any therapist ever could in a matter of an hour or so. A hypnotherapist engaging in effective roles (investigator and co-creator), getting clients to trust their unconscious mind—that they *do* have the answers, is going to increase the hypnotherapist's success rate. Trusting the unconscious may be done by simply asking the client, "What do you need me to tell your subconscious mind?" or "Does this suggestion sound good to you?" and getting verbal or nonverbal agreement. With enough hands-on practice, we become observant enough to notice that the client will "light up," as I refer, when the right suggestion is rehearsed with the client during the interview. When this happens, it indicates that this is a good suggestion to write down and utilize later when the client is under trance.

The client interview methods discussed, and the individualized suggestive scripting techniques, may be used either independently as the primary method of intervention during each hypnotherapy session, or they can be used in conjunction with other suggestive therapies, such as scripts or imagery techniques. When first starting out to practice hypnotherapy, sometimes we will find the need to spend a little extra time pondering what suggestion best fits our client; but with time and experience, we will learn to simply trust the unconscious for the best way to proceed.

Chapter 17

Hypnotic Regression

Hypnotic regression is perhaps the single most powerful intervention for creating a change in an individual's character in the shortest amount of time, while it increases awareness about the self and our world like nothing else on earth; and it does so not only through new understandings, consciously, but also experientially and unconsciously. Since the roots of our character are unconscious, and hypnotic regression illuminates these roots, clients of regression can change the programming that exists from the past instantaneously. Once this illumination occurs, through the assistance of the more mature current state of consciousness of the client, and the effect of two minds being better than one (the input of the hypnotherapist), a highly effective healing which lasts a lifetime often takes place. With these two variables, old memory files can be updated and turned into new memory files. What I sometimes tell my clients is, "The red memory files get updated and put into the blue memory files."

New hypnotherapists, and their clients, often wonder how regression therapy compares to suggestive therapy, in getting results. Which one is best to use and when? I tell them that suggestive therapy is just as powerful, but in a more subtle way. Suggestive therapy is a lot more comfortable for the client, and in many cases it is easier on the hypnotherapist as well. No hypnotherapist is required to use regression therapy. In fact, there are some in the field that exclusively use suggestive therapy and are still very busy with regular clientele. Yet, the power of hypnotic regression cannot be ignored, particularly since clients will spontaneously regress, from time to time, during suggestive therapy sessions. For that reason, it is beneficial for students of hypnotherapy to at least have introductory training in hypnotic regression, in order to be able to recognize it and respond when it does occur.

The golden rule

The golden rule that I practice under for selecting an intervention, whether to use suggestive therapy or hypnotic regression therapy, is a follows:

Use suggestive therapy, unless the client calls for regression.

A client could call the hypnotherapist's office and simply ask to be regressed. This occurs as a result of reoccurring nightmares, negative memories, the desire to do some personal growth or spiritual exploration, embrace the wounded child for therapeutic purposes, or to simply remember something from the past that has been forgotten. The reasons for regression are practically endless. Sometimes, a client may not be responding to suggestive therapy after one or two sessions. It is at that point that I discuss finding the causative factors which may exist in the unconscious mind's memory bank. If the client is willing, then we have nothing to lose by trying this method, and in many cases much to gain. In addition to instant healing, sometimes a regression gives us more information we can use to formulate suggestions to be given to the client at the end of the session or on a subsequent session.

Memories and The Brain

The concept that the brain held forgotten memories was documented by Karl Pribram. In his research, he worked with a woman who had a hole in her skull, so that her brain could be safely stimulated with a probe. One day, when he stimulated a neurological pathway, she had a vivid memory of age two.

In effect, he proved that memories are forgotten, or unconscious, but yet are stored neurologically in the brain, where they may still affect us. This experiment may also describe how hypnotic regression takes place on a physiological level. Perhaps the neural pathways get stimulated through hypnosis, which can produce unconscious memories. Yet, this scientific explanation does not accurately describe how Cayce accessed the memories of his clients, so we must include the metaphysical (or nonphysical) component of memory, which is Mind, and accurately state that the mind is non-local. It is not limited to physiological boundaries. Based on these concepts, we could speculate that memories can originate from either the brain or the mind, or perhaps both at the same time.

Associated vs. Dissociated Trance:

Although previously mentioned in this text, we will review associated and dissociated states, in reference to hypnotic regression:

Associated means to be completely associated into an experience that is being encountered under hypnosis. When a client is associated into a memory, he or she tends to experience reliving, often using present tense wording as if going through it again (e.g. "I am...").

Dissociated describes an experience in which a client is detached when describing his or her experience. When a client is dissociated in a memory, he or she experiences memory recall, often using past tense wording (e.g. "I was...").

Generally, a deep level trance characterizes an associated memory experience, while a lighter trance characterizes a dissociated memory experience. Associated memories bring about stronger feelings and more details, while dissociated memories bring about the opposite, less feelings and less detail. A client undergoing regression will sometimes experience the effect of being associated one minute and dissociated the next. Throughout the session, many clients experience intermittently going deeper and lighter into the memory experience.

Some hypnotherapists prefer the client to be dissociated, so that they do not relive any of the emotions that may be triggered by memory regression. They contend that when it comes to negative memory experiences, once is enough; the client need not go through the feelings all over again. They also contend that just making the unconscious information conscious restores healing and balance. Reframing the memory is most important.

Other hypnotherapists prefer for the client to be more associated. This group contends that catharsis is more effective because it purifies the emotions, which are held in the neuromuscular system of the body. Once released, there is increased health and a deeper sense of peace and harmony.

Either method is effective in achieving therapeutic goals, and depends on the preferences of the client and therapist. Some hypnotherapists negotiate how a regression may be experienced before the regression session, others negotiate only upon encountering strong emotions. I am generally of the latter practice, but sometimes have discussed the possible effect of regression, in regards to a potential catharsis, with some clients who have shown concern in the past.

Another term for hypnotic regression is *age regression*. This term originated from an effect that Pierre Janet discovered in the middle of the twentieth century, when he was Freud's student. He found that his clients could mentally regress to younger ages when put under hypnosis. *Revivification,* or reliving, was found to take place when someone was undergoing a deeper more associated state of hypnosis, such as in age regression. In regression, there is a part of the mind that feels as if it is reliving the memory, while another part of the mind stays conscious and aware of the present moment to discuss the memory with a hypnotherapist.

Regression Procedures

1) Interview:

When it has been discussed and decided upon, or the hypnotherapist and the client agree that hypnotic regression would be a good method to try, discussing *expectation* would be the next step. If the client has undergone a regression in the past, then he or she knows what to expect and less preparation is necessary. If the client has not undergone a regression before, the following step is recommended.

Car/House imaginability test:

With this test, we are priming the subconscious mind and helping the client discover what regression is. This is done by asking the client to remember what his or her car or house looks like. This only takes a few seconds. Then the client acknowledges that he or she has it, by saying "OK," or something like that. The hypnotherapist then asks what angle they are seeing it from, and the client usually, if they have any ability to visually image, responds with seeing it from the front, side, back, or from inside.

At that point the other primary sensory channels are included by asking the client what he or she hears and feels. The more information the client describes, the more lifelike the memory becomes. It is important to bring this to the client's attention. The hypnotherapist can then emphasize how the images were selected randomly by the subconscious mind, and the more the client described them, the more clear they became. All this started by trusting the subconscious. Trusting that whatever is brought to an individual's awareness is exactly what we are looking for. Often, there will be something significant about the specific room in the house, or something about the car, that the subconscious focused on. It should be brought to the client's attention that this is because the subconscious mind selects that which is most important about the subject matter at the current time.

It is important that an analogy be drawn between this memory and a hypnotic memory. The only difference is that a memory under hypnosis appears to be more vivid. Because a client will often doubt forgotten memories, since they surface from the unconscious mind and are not readily recognized consciously, it is often important to help the client trust whatever the subconscious mind brings up during the session. The client is the filter for such experiences, describing the information that he or she is experiencing to the hypnotherapist.

2) Induction:

It is good to use a formal psychophysical induction method. At the point right before regressing the client, it is advisable to use 2 or 3 deepening techniques. This helps the unconscious and subconscious mind areas to be more active, and it increases the likelihood that a regression method will be successful in accessing subconscious information, as opposed to conscious information. Even with two or three deepening techniques, generally because the new client knows that an activity will be required of them, and he or she is inquisitive or excited, only a medium state of hypnosis is usually achieved. Medium levels of hypnosis work well for regression, but once a client undergoes hypnosis more than once, deeper levels that lead to revivification are generally achieved.

3) Implement a Regression Method:

There are three primary regression classifications. Most regression methods fall under more than one of the following categories:

a) Reorientation:

This is where the client is asked to imagine that his or her mind or consciousness is leaving the present moment and moving back into the dimensions of mind where it stores the past. Imagery tools tend to be involved for imagining this time-travel experience. The client imagines leaving the present and reorienting to the past.

b) Descending Order:

In the early days of regression, the hypnotist used birthdays to regress the client. The birthdays of each year were remembered, one year at a time, until the year was reached that would contain pertinent information. In later years, imagery tools were used to imagine going back through, or over, the years. Sometimes the hypnotherapist sets up a continuum of years and asks the client to imagine going over specific ages.

c) Open Ended:
Dr. Irene Hickman, who wrote *Mind Probe Hypnosis*, made this method popular. She would put the client under hypnosis and ask him or her to simply, "Go back to the source of the problem." After a brief period of waiting, the cause of the problem was usually discovered in the form of a memory. Then, the client was asked to describe the story which the subconscious brought forward, and which contained the problem.

Regression Scripts

Scripts are the easiest way to begin using regression. The following are a few regression scripts that I've extracted from another book that I have written, mentioned earlier, titled, *Script Magic: A Hypnotherpist's Desk Reference*. Notice that the scripts use all combinations of the classifications of regression tools: reorientation, descending order, and open ended.

Count Back Regression:
"OK, now I want you to imagine which direction your subconscious mind stores the past. Your past memories could be located above you, beside you, in front or behind you. I want you to allow yourself to float back into that direction now, leaving the present behind... I will count from one to five, and I want you to allow yourself to float back over as many years as is necessary to find (state the goal). One... leaving the present and floating back toward the direction of the past. Two... floating back over the years. Three... farther back and more deeply relaxed. Four... approaching the (goal)...and you're there now at the number Five."

Time Tunnel Regression:
(To be done at the end of the stairs deepening technique.)
"At the end of the stairs there's a doorway marked "Memories." When you open the doorway there is a long tunnel with a light at the end of it symbolizing birth. You begin to walk down the tun-

nel and there are windows from different scenes of your life. In the windows, you notice yourself as being younger and younger. You may go back as far as is necessary for (state the goal). You will either float through a window or float through the bright light at the end of the tunnel and you will be there. When I count from one to five, you will be there. One...two...three...four...five."

Open Ended Regression:

"When I count from one to five, you will go back to the cause of the problem. Simply trust whatever your subconscious mind brings you. Whatever it shows you will be the source of the problem. One...two...three...four...five."

Other Regression Techniques

Time Line Regression:

This is where individuals float above a time line, which is perceived as a linear representation of all of his or her memories, or unique path through time. He or she then floats back toward the past section of the time line and into a segment that contains a pertinent memory.

Forest-Garden Paths:

The client imagines a beautiful garden in the middle of a forest. There is a spirit guide there that takes the client down a path that will lead to the most important memory.

Affect Bridge Regression:

This tool is used with clients that are already generally familiar with regression. The client locates a feeling in the body, and then he or she is asked to simply go back to the first time he or she first felt that way.

Advanced Regression Techniques

Once the hypnotherapist regresses the client into a perti-nent memory, there are other tools that will help increase the level of content and clarity. These are tools that are to be used after a regression method is performed and a memory begins to surface within the client's subconscious mind:

1) Hypnoanalysis questions:

These questions are open-ended because this encourages the client to focus on the content which is taking place in the mind's eye. Closed-ended questions are often less effective, because they might start a set of "no"s. Erickson recommended getting the client in a "yes-set," so that resistance would be reduced and the subconscious mind would be more responsive.

a. "What are you aware of?"
b. "What's happening?"
c. "What happens next?"
d. "And then what happens?"
e. "What else are you aware of?"

2) Locating the Initial Sensitizing Event:

Locating the most important memory, with the most rel-evant information, is the goal of regression therapy. This can be done by simply asking the client to... "Move forward to the next significant event." In most cases, once the client is regressed he or she is already there, but if the session is not turning up any significant information, the suggestion above will lead to the most significant event, where most of the therapeutic transformation will likely take place. It is believed that once the initial sensitizing event is encountered in a regression, a paradigm shift will occur, changing relative patterns of memories that occurred thereafter, through the present, and into the future.

3) 4x/90-10 rule:

I developed this rule for new hypnotherapists, so that there would be a better understanding of how clients behave under hypnosis, and hypnotherapists may adjust their own methods accordingly. One rule that stands true for most hypnotic regression sessions is that the client's mind is experiencing thoughts four times (4x) slower than the hypnotherapist's mind. Therefore, it is important to pause and wait for the client to gather information and answer one question before asking another. This pause, or silence, will often last anywhere from 10 seconds to 2 minutes, depending on how much information the client is divulging.

The tendency for the new hypnotherapist is to rush the client into talking by zinging him or her with a series of questions, before he or she has a chance to answer. This is commonly very disturbing for the client. The client needs the pauses or gaps in conversation, in order to allow the slow moving imagery to unfold. Then, the client can express all of the details of his or her experience, one segment at a time.

Another portion of this rule is that the client is experiencing about 90% more information than what he or she is able to tell the hypnotherapist while in the altered state. In other words, the therapist is only privileged to about 10% of what the client is experiencing. For this reason, hypnoanalysis oriented questions are best, with a good dose of patience. At the end of the session, during the post session interview, the client may or may not feel like discussing more of the details, but if so, it may prove to be the best place to be updated. The key is to know enough about what is going on to facilitate the session.

Another portion of this rule is that the client's voice is only going to be at about 10% of the normal volume. Some clients sound like they are whispering, while others simply talk very softly, slurring their words. To the client, it sounds like he or she is talking at regular volume, because of the hyper-awareness phenomena associated with hypnosis. It may be difficult for the hypnotherapist to hear what the client is saying, so he or she might need to move closer to the client. Another method is to have the client wear a lavaliere microphone to where the hypnotherapist may amplify the voice and record it at the same time. Yet, in most cases, if it is reasonably quiet in the office, the client will still be able to be adequately heard.

One client-type that generally does not fit this rule is the visually dominant client who is in a lighter to medium trance. In this case, the client tends to talk more normally, describing more details.

Handling Resistance to Regression

There are a few common resistances to regression that may be encountered that are worth discussing in the following paragraphs. The primary variable that determines a good regression client involves conditioning. If the client has undergone altered states of consciousness before, he or she is destined to do well. If not, it may be best to get a self-hypnosis tape to the client before the session. If this is not possible, and it is the clients first altered state experience, a long formal induction, with two to three deepening techniques, may increase susceptibility and reduce potential resistance. When examining the proper responses to resistances below, it is important to keep in mind that patience on the part of the hypnotherapist is the key to overcoming most resistances.

A) The client opens his or her eyes:

Clients are still under hypnosis when they open their eyes, even though they often do not think so. Additionally, what occurs is much the same as compound suggestion. This is where the client is brought in and out of trance until the conscious mind becomes confused. Then, a much greater depth of hypnosis is achieved.

Response= "If you close your eyes, you'll be able to concentrate better. Each time you open and close your eyes, you will go deeper."

B) The client's response is "Nothing.":

When asked the hypnoanalysis questions mentioned previously, clients may respond that they are aware of "nothing." It may be that the sensory modalities surfacing in the memory are not consistent with the semantic suggestion of the hypnotherapist. In other words, the hypnotherapist may be asking the client what he or she "sees." If the client is in the 25% of the population that has a low visual sensory mode, he or she may actually be less able to visualize. So it is important to use the words, "What are you *aware* of?" or a question that does not limit the senses by implying a particular sensory channel.

Sometimes, the client is afraid to encounter something emotionally painful, so even though the individual is experiencing a memory, he or she is not willing to tell the hypnotherapist about it. Sometimes the hypnotherapist should reconsider rapport. Perhaps it would be best to further discuss the goal or intent behind regression, before attempting another regression session.

Sometimes the client may not be trusting imagery that he or she is experiencing. In other words, the client has very clear images of something that he or she does not recognize, which is often the case when experiencing forgotten memories.

Response= Try and try again

1) Choosing a memory for the client:
Sometimes the hypnotherapist may simply choose a memory for the client, such as the first time he or she rode a bicycle, or played on a playground. If the client can not remember these easily enough, then it may be that the client is expecting something that simply will not take place. Perhaps the client expects to fall asleep, or become completely detached from the present. Once a memory is accessed, then other memories should come more easily.

2) Consciously thinking too much:
If the client seems to be a very rational person, with a strong left-brain dominance, a confusion method of sorts may be attempted, such as those discussed previously in this book. This will reduce the conscious mind's activity. Reframing the conscious mind, which is also listed in the chapter on deepening, is another good tool for these client-types.

3) Take them into deeper trance level:
Sometimes the client is not in a deep enough trance level for the unconscious mind to start producing imagery. In that case, one or two more deepening techniques may be applied. These can be repeated after attempting a regression while the client is still under hypnosis.

Regressive-Transformational Models

Once memory content begins to emerge, the therapist should spend an adequate amount of time gathering information through a lengthy period of open-ended questions. The following models may be applied near the end of the session by the more experienced hypnotherapist.

1. Desensitization-

This process was first used by Irene Hickman in her book *Mind Probe Hypnosis*. It involves rerunning an emotionally loaded memory from beginning to end, until all of the emotion is gone and the client is desensitized. After repeating the memory several times, a catharsis, or sense of purification occurs, and present-day triggers are dissolved. Afterward, the client may reexamine the memory consciously, and he or she feels neutral. This method is ideal for past-life or abstract regressions, as it stimulates detail. It is also a good choice for eliminating fears and phobias. It is, however, in my opinion, contraindicated for childhood trauma recovery, as this form of associated abreaction may be too overpowering.

2. Differentiation-

After developing and fine-tuning this technique, I found it to be effective not only for habit triggers but any patterns that the client may find themselves in, from any time of existence. This technique involves the client reviewing the *past* memory under hypnosis and examining the *present* problem simultaneously and asking the client, "What's similar between the past and present? (pause for the answer). Now, what's different between the past and present?" This model can be used effectively in abstract regression whereby the client is asked to compare the "past life" to the present life. Also, this model is ideal for dissolving unhealthy past beliefs, or habit triggers, (e.g. starvation experienced in a person's childhood means he or she should eat more food in the present, in order to eliminate starvation from occurring again). Differentiation is primarily used to update the unconscious mind with current, logical realizations.

3. Soul Retrieval-

This model is ideal for those who do not feel a sense of wholeness, or feel as if a part of themselves is missing. These methods were originally developed by Sandra Ingerman, who wrote the book, *Soul Retrieval: Mending the Fragmented Self*. She wrote information on the Native American and shamanic healing process known as "soul retrieval." In shamanism, the practitioner finds the fragmented self within his or her own imagery, and then informs the client of the recovery. In hypnosis, the rituals are eliminated and the retrieval process is performed by the client and facilitated by the therapist, as opposed to the other way around. This process is done by having the client regress and remember a time where they were whole or possessed a desired talent. This method is good to use for childhood briefest trauma recovery in place of, or in addition to, wounded child blending. I most commonly use this model at the end of a series of wounded child sessions when I work with psychological referrals.

4. Wounded Child Blending-

Originally, this concept came from such books as, *Healing The Child Within*, by Charles Whitfield, and *Homecoming*, by John Bradshaw. It was designed for people who felt inadequacies that stemmed from a dysfunctional childhood. Wounded child therapists have often been known to tell their clients that their wounded child may be doing the work for their adult self. The more difficult the childhood was, generally the more fragmented a person may feel in everyday life.

The aforementioned wounded-child, or inner-child, pioneers began by having their clients imagine that their adult-selves were going back to a place where their wounded child existed within their subconscious mind. Upon discovering the inner-child, the client was to embrace or reparent that part of their consciousness. These memories, when utilized in hypnotic regression, tend to be powerful fragmentation-blending experiences. It is best for hypnotherapists to dissociate the client, having them rise above such memories, so that the memory is experienced in a more dissociated fashion (remembering the memory from the present perspective).

This proves to be more comfortable for the client, than if he or she was fully associated into the memory.

5. Higher-Self or Spirit Guidance-

In this model, a higher self, spirit guide, or angel, is accessed for use during the session. A higher-self is often perceived by the client as a higher part of him or herself that contains answers to various problems. The higher-self is often referred to as part of the unconscious mind, while angels and spirit guides are generally perceived as being of a higher-power with answers that are from outside of, but connected to, the self. These guides may be perceived as part of the superconscious mind. The label given for this effect will depend on the belief structure of the client. Once this dimension of reality is accessed, this third party effect can be asked to lead the session to the most productive memory for the client. After the memories are accessed, this force can be called upon for a final opinion at the end of the session.

New hypnotherapists may find this highly useful as a third party does all of the counseling to transform the problem. The drawback may be that the hypnotherapist occasionally has difficlties finding a guide, angel, or higher-self to assist the session. Sometimes it is easier to find a higher-self than an angel or spirit guide. Many times it takes a lengthy amount of time, and a deep trance level, to find such entities.

6. Visual Emotional Clearing-

This is a process whereby there is very little or no catharsis involved. It requires that the client is somewhat visual, and it is very good for those clients who are not comfortable with experiencing their emotions. Although catharsis is circumvented, this method still tends to be very effective. Once the memory is accessed, the client is asked to see the emotion in the memory like a dark cloud of metallic dust, which can be picked up with a magnet that the present self holds above the memory. Then the big black ball is pulled off of the end of the magnet and thrown out into space until it burns up in the sun. This form of therapy can be very effective for veterans of war, and other traumatized individuals.

7. Trust the Unconscious-

This statement is derived from Doctor Milton Erickson. When applied to hypnotic regression, it is an approach that facilitates the client's memories to emerge. In many sessions, clients may not know exactly where they are in the memory process and why they are there; but once they are encouraged to "trust your unconscious" (memory imagery), rather than discard a foreign image, they will often embrace it and more detail can emerge. Sometimes clients switch from one scene to the next and the hypnotherapist must simply keep up with what the client is experiencing. In these cases, it is impossible to run the client through a transformational model. We must follow the client wherever they go within themselves until they tire and awaken or request to be counted out of hypnosis.

The above transformational models have been expanded upon, with detailed step-by-step procedures and scripts, in a work I wrote and titled the *Master Manual*. In addition to the transformational models mentioned, other models are expounded upon, and some models have submodels, or alternative procedures depending on the memory type. Because of the sensitive (soul-level) material that surfaces during sessions, it is my belief that further training beyond this text is essential for those that are interested in specializing in hypnotic regression therapy. At the time of writing and revising this book, the master manual was currently only available to students of my master program; however, a text that is a spin-off from the master manual is underway and should be released soon.

In the meantime, I feel that the best way to become acquainted with regression is to perform abstract regressions, or what I refer to as "past-life exploration." These memories are further away from home, figuratively speaking, and give the student of hypnotherapy a base to work from and discover if this area of hypnotherapy is suited to them. In the chapter on abstract regression, I will mention books that are ideal for beginning a study of this exploratory and therapeutic process.

Determining the Transformational Model

The choice of the transformational model is best determined by the client's belief structure, the level of rapport developed, the client's previous experience with therapy, and the goal of hypnotherapy:

A) Client-type and belief structure:
It is best to operate within a client's belief structure. This expedites results (instead of the client encountering states of confusion), and increases our success rate (due to the loss of rapport if we are not client centered). For example, if a client believes in angels and that he or she can access them under hypnosis, then we can utilize this particular model with a high degree of success. If the client does not believe in angels, but believes there is a higher part of him or herself that can provide the answer to specific problems, then that is what the hypnotherapist should utilize for obtaining the best results. Although encountering angels, and other dimensional realities, are often very enlightening and transformative, we tend to waste time on unwilling converts!

B) Rapport:
With greater rapport, a client can be more easily influenced to experience new models of transformation. For example, I remember a client who was not inclined to believe in angels, but when asked her if she wanted to encounter one to help us solve her night eating problems, she agreed. It took us a long time to access her guide, but once we did so, the guide took us to a memory when she was in her late twenties (she was in her sixties at the time) and had been hospitalized for a severe ulcer. The hospital staff woke her up during the night to eat a pasty, unsatisfying substance, leaving her hungry for normal food.
After the session, she recovered from the problem. However, she would have never even attempted such a regression had she not had two sessions of suggestive therapy prior, when the rapport was very solid.

C) Client's previous experience with therapy:
A client's previous experience with therapy will have a

direct effect on what they expect the hypnotherapist to provide them in solving their problems. If a client has come as a referral from a mental health group that specializes in wounded child therapy, he or she will come to expect this type of work. Childhood memory therapy will likely be where the client gravitates under regression. It is logical to consider expectation when clients come in for regression therapy or exploration. Their prior exposure to therapy, or hypnotherapy (TV, word of mouth, etc.) will often set the stage for their regressive experiences.

D. Goal of hypnotherapy:

The goal a client brings into private practice in the beginning of therapy should always be acted upon, as a general rule. If the client comes in to quit smoking, and we tell him or her that he or she is too depressed or stressed to quit (based on information in the first interview), and we advise the client to do regression or start a stress management program before attempting to quit smoking, we are likely to limit his or her results or lose the client all together. If we act upon the momentum that a client brings into a session to begin with, we are more likely to be successful.

It is always best to stay client centered, and goal oriented. In effective hypnotherapy, the goals are always set by the client beforehand, and then the hypnotherapist manages those goals with the client. This management system is a negotiation process that determines the number of sessions that are needed in most cases. When the goals which the client set for themselves in the beginning are met, hypnotherapy generally terminates.

Two Things that Create Functional and Dysfunctional Behavior

1. An objective physical, external event.

2. The resulting-subjective mental, physical and emotional internal representation, or perceptual awareness, during and after the event.

Every individual is left with perceptual realities from each experience they have had in the past, and these are purely subjective. Although an objective and concrete experience occurred, a subjective experience is the result during and after the event. Therefore, it is most important that the hypnotherapist have the ability to share the client's perceptions to the point of developing empathy. If the therapist cannot share the client's perceptions to that point, empathy may be lacking, and the therapy is likely to lack effectiveness. The therapist should imagine that they are a lawyer representing the client's case or perceptions. If the hypnotherapist cannot represent their client's perceptions, he or she may be better off referring the case to other therapists, which would benefit both parties.

A certain level of empathy is required to be effective, but a level of detachment is also necessary to survive any helping profession. As a result, all helping professionals need to strike a balance between the two for sustaining their ideals and purpose in their profession, and in their personal lives as well.

Personality Formation

To get a better understanding of the subconscious selection process, which utilizes beliefs and values to create meaning in the material world, it is important to understand that the subconscious mind always selects what it intends to be the most efficient and effective thought, emotion, and/or behavior in every moment. Although this process does not always bring about the intended outcome, we can still embrace the agenda of the unconscious mind, and understand that problematic feelings and behaviors are being selected for a greater purpose. This purpose is for us to embrace our significant life experiences, or as Carl Jung often referred, "our shadows." In doing this, we become enlightened. It is many of these most significant experiences that form personality.

For a greater understanding at this natural subconscious selection process, let's look at the work of the Sociologist Morris Massey. He theorized that human beings have *significant life experiences*, (S.L.E.s), during the years of personality formation from birth through age 21. These determine their current day behaviors. He referred to the time period of birth through age seven as the "imprint" stage of personality formation. Here, significant life experiences during that age span are permanently imprinted upon our personality. Age eight through 13 is considered the "modeling" stage, where we model important others, and age 14 to 21 is referred to as the "socialization" stage, where we socialize our personality to near completion.

According to Massey, it is the S.L.E.s, most of which occurred before the age of eight, which serve as determining factors in our unconsciously driven behaviors, in addition to the structure of our beliefs and values. These tend to drive emotions, which then tend to drive behaviors. As a result, if the client brings out a problematic S.L.E., either consciously (during the interview) or unconsciously (while under hypnosis), it often creates substantial positive changes in the long term.

Dr. Chips' Core Values Grid

Over the years, I have conducted several thousand sessions in hypnotherapy. These sessions were in a wide variety of settings. The client's goals have varied widely, and so have their value systems. I've observed a variety of attitude, belief, and value structures, through the study and practice of transpersonal hypnotherapy. It appears that those clients who had expressed a higher power component as a perceptual reality within their lives often felt self-empowered after hypnotherapy interventions and were able to progress more quickly. They were able to look at adversity as that which occurred to assist them in becoming a greater being, while those with negative beliefs about themselves and others, which were often driven from their residual perceptions regarding past vulnerabilities, progressed more slowly through the therapeutic change process, as well as through life itself. The following core values grid that I created helps predict a client's progress relative to the speed and the effectiveness of a healing or transformation.

Core Values Grid

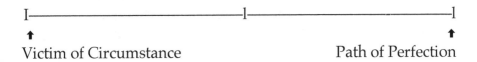

I———————————————I———————————————I
↑   ↑
Victim of Circumstance   Path of Perfection

As the reader reflects on the values grid, he or she will notice that there are two extreme individuals at each end, for the purpose of education. The grid emphasizes core values or what is transpersonally referred to as the client's spiritual orientation. An extreme on one end of the grid is the individual who lacks a good concept of a higher-power. This person has a "victim of circumstance" awareness. It means that no matter what happens in life, he or she ends up being the victim. Life just happens to these people and they are therefore at the "effect" end of "cause and effect" or life's occurrences. Many of these clients progress very slowly and often will give up their self-power to their therapist so to put the therapist at *cause* and leave themselves at *effect*. Only the very experienced hypnotherapist should work with these client-types, and preferably those with advanced levels of education.

If a hypnotherapist works with a client longer than just a few sessions, they may start encountering the client's deeper values and discover that the client is at the lower end of the grid. If so, the client may be encouraged to make a spiritual connection, thereby raising their location on the values grid. Thus, he or she becomes an easier client, less taxing on the hypnotherapist, and is happier with change, and life in general.

At the opposite end of the grid is the individual that believes that everything that happens in life involves his or her higher-power relationship. Somehow there is a purpose behind every experience, or a higher reason. If this purpose is not immediately revealed, it will eventually come to light to make all experiences part of the "path of perfection." Individuals on this end of the grid tend to include what higher-source experience had led them to the hypnotherapist, as well as what transpires during and after therapy as a result of the intention of their higher-power. These individuals are self-empowered during and after therapy and therefore often feel that the hypnotherapist is simply another stepping stone in the master plan. Their place in the greater scheme of life unfolds at an appropriate rate. Often, the most rewarding clients to work with are those whose core value is high on the path of perfection.

Most individuals fall somewhere in the middle of the values grid, due to the completely unique variables in the form of past experiences that are stored in the unconscious mind. In addition to subconscious programming, it is the will, ego, or conscious selection process that organizes an individual's values into a uniquely intricate and logical perceptual sequence. In other words, each individual attaches various perceptual values to his or her subconscious selections. Therefore, how "functional" or "dysfunctional" an experience was, is determined by the perceptual values an individual places on those memory representations.

Using transformational models is a good way to get started in regression therapy and begin getting positive results. It is also recommended that hypnotherapists experience regression from the client's perspective, so that there is a deeper understanding of how the process of change actually takes place through this particular methodology. There are many ways to continue further training in regression therapy. One way to do so is to contact the association listed in the afterword of this text and inquire about a program in close proximity to home, or that which can be traveled to for an intensive training over a number of days. Another way to learn is experientially, by finding instances where clients present opportunities to utilize these transformative models.

There are a number of ways for new hypnotherapists to "get their feet wet," in order to experience one of the most powerful methods available today for creating profound and lasting changes. The keys for deciding to embark upon such an inner journey involves the hypnotherapist's readiness and the synchronistic aspect of the clients who present themselves to try such an approach.

Chapter 18

Abstract Regression

Because "past-life" memories are less tangible than current life memories, and it is important to stay client-centered, not advocating beliefs one way or another, I refer to this section as abstract regression. This enables us to take a non-biased approach and perhaps embrace the therapeutic value of this phenomenon. People that embrace these images as memories from their past-lives generally believe in reincarnation. However, there are other explanations for this phenomenon that we can explore. Likewise, hypnotherapists should keep an open mind and not exclude the many cases of accurately researched past-lives that indicate the authenticity that human beings, at least some, have the ability to reincarnate. Assuming that we are spiritual beings, who are created from an unlimited source, or God, then anything is possible. Philosophy aside, we will primarily focus on the therapeutic benefits of this form of regression therapy, as most of us are not researchers but are involved in this work because we are therapists.

There are three primary explanations for abstract regressions/past-life memories, that are important for the student of hypnotherapy to consider, before committing to specific beliefs.

Three Primary Explanations
for the "Past-life" Phenomenon

1) One Life Position:

This position is often held by skeptics who believe that we live only one life. The mind is blank slate at birth. What is referred to as past-life phenomena might be a result of cryptoamnesia, genetic memory, possession, or confabulation.

Cryptoamnesia is where a child's unconscious mind may have recorded information with dates, places, etc., from the media or stories. When he or she reaches adulthood and undergoes a hypnotic regression, the details of the past-life memory may not be what it appears to be. Instead, it may be information from a movie that his or her unconscious mind recorded and is reproducing under hypnosis.

Some fundamentalist or conservative religious types who share this view believe this phenomenon is a result of possession. It is hypothesized by some that a dead person's soul is roaming the earth, so that when a person undergoes hypnosis, he or she becomes opened up to possession. At that time, the dead person speaks through the living person's body and expresses the memories of the life that they spent on earth. Although this theory is less popular lately, it still exists in some circles.

Genetic memory is another explanation, which maintains that it is possible that what is considered to be past-life memories are actually the memories of our ancestors. Through our genes, these memories are transferred to the brain and can later come out in a state of hypnosis. This theory is gaining in popularity, under the one life position.

Metaphors, or confabulation, is another explanation under this position, where an individual creates faces and situations for his or her complexities of current day life. These complexes play themselves out, such as in a dream.

2) Collective Unconscious Position:

Carl Jung often referred to the *collective unconscious* as a place where all humans are connected to each other in consciousness. It is a place, he thought, that is responsible for our intuitive abilities, dreams, and more.

Edgar Cayce referred to this same area as the *supercon-scious*. It was believed that he could access this place by spiraling up through the super conscious mind to find the akashic records and past-life memories of various individuals who requested his readings.

Under this position, it is possible that a hypnotized individual could remember the life of any other person while under hypnosis. If this is possible, then the lives that some individuals are recalling under hypnosis may not necessarily be their own.

To further emphasize this ability in a hypnotized individual, an author by the name of Dolores Cannon has written several books on putting people under hypnosis and researching the collective unconscious. In her research, she accesses and reinterprets the lives and prophecies of Nostradamus and Christ. This position may explain why so many people who have undergone past-life regression have thought themselves to have lived the life of Joan of Ark; instead, they may actually be accessing her memories from the collective unconscious rather than their own unconscious mind. How this exactly takes place under hypnosis is further expounded upon in the chapter on "The Cayce Effect."

3) The Reincarnation Position:

This position claims that reincarnation is indeed plausible. It indicates that there is a universal conscious forgetting process at our birth that enables people to forget why they have entered into earthly existence. Yet, unconscious memory still exists and it determines where we synchronistically incarnate, which scenarios we engage in, and with whom we spend our lives.

Philosophically speaking, knowledge and wisdom is gained through each incarnation, which results in character growth and eventually enlightenment. Karma, which is defined by eastern religions as "carry over" from one life to the next, governs the fate of each individual in each incarnation. Karma is consistent with the western biblical view that, what we sow, we shall reap. Good deeds return to us as pleasurable events, and bad deeds return to us as painful events.

There are many documented and convincing cases for past-life memories. Research is being shown on the major television networks of our era, demonstrating how several individuals have gotten names, dates, and places while under hypnosis, and later documented their actual existence. Many people have also spontaneously remembered past-lifetimes that have existed on the earth, without hypnosis. There are many cases where Ian Stevenson, PhD, at the University of Virginia, documented the memories of young children having lived on the earth before. Some research suggests that children who speak foreign languages, without any exposure to them, have remembered lifetimes in foreign countries. The National Association of Transpersonal Hypnotherapists (NATH), listed in the Afterword of this book, has several documented cases of reincarnation on video tape that are quite impressive. These remain the property of the association and are sometimes shown at various conference locations. In addition, it is quite possible that our local library carries some of the most popular researched cases of reincarnation.

For those students of hypnotherapy who desire a working knowledge of past-life regression research, exploration, and therapy, I recommend the books, *Life Patterns, Soul Lessons & Forgiveness*, and *The Journey Within: Past-life Regression and Channeling*, both by Henry Leo Bolduc. These may be accessed on the publisher's page in the back of this book.

"Past-life" Illustrations

When considering the purpose of reincarnation, the reader should consider two primary sources that were invaluable in teaching and understanding such concepts. The first is Buddha, and the second is Edgar Cayce. Buddha's teachings, with several hundred individual past-life regressions I've conducted, are from where I've drawn most to create past-life theory A; and Edgar Cayce is the second source I've accessed for creating past-life theory B.

In the first illustration, *Past-life Theory-A*, we can see the tree of life as being a metaphor for past-life influences on the current life. Buddha was once asked by one of his students how many past-lives the common person has. Buddha was laying under a

Past Life Theory-A

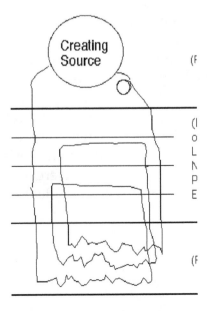

Past Life Theory-B

large tree at the time, and he was said to point up into its branches and claim that the answer was in the number of leaves that were in the tree.

For metaphorical purposes, let's imagine that the roots are past-life factors for the trunk of the tree, which is where a person incarnates into the earth plane. The individual can go through transition (die) at any point within a predetermined set of outcomes for that life. Free-will determines how well the individual does, and therefore where he ends up. At the end of the life cycle, the individual comes back to the superconscious area or astral plane (represented by the falling leaf), where another incarnation may be planned, if deemed necessary.

The second illustration, *Past-life Theory-B,* was taken from Cayce readings which indicated that the primary goal of a human being is to master the cycle of rebirth. In essence, once the individual reaches a certain point in spiritual evolution, there is no need to continue to be reborn. The illustration shows a process of becoming more like our creator, which may be a primary purpose behind reincarnation. This may explain why the western biblical text states, "The goal is to be perfect like your Father in heaven." Christ also states that, "Elijah has returned. You know him as John the Baptist" and "You must be born again to enter into the kingdom of heaven." Perhaps these passages indicate the cycle of rebirth and becoming more like our creator, until which point we return to the creator.

In his readings, Cayce described how all souls must return to source, some with a name and some without a name. If this is true, then we must ponder what having a name, or separate identity, means, in regards to being human and returning home. In addition, it may be interesting to hypothesize what it means for souls that return to source without a name, or identity. I often ponder this reading and illustration in reference to self-love. Perhaps if we love the self, we return with an identity, and if we hate the self we do not.

Abstract Residues

In order to comprehend the full extent of which past-life therapy encompasses, we will want to consider residues. It is residues that determine carry-over from one life to the next. Karma is often found in the physical, mental, and emotional dimensions of our client. These often serve as spring boards, or windows, into past-life regressions, when appropriately utilized as such in the interview. Past-life therapists have been known to state, "What has been done in the physical, must be undone in the physical," when referring to karmic carry-overs that dictate circumstances in the current life.

a. <u>Physical</u> residues may show up as birth marks on the physical body. A person's physical illnesses or diseases may also be indicative of past-life residue (e.g. an ulcer clears up after a client remembers a past-life where he got stabbed in the side with a sword).
b. <u>Mental</u> residues can be found in the client's perceptions. Current life values and generalizations may be a result of mental residues carried over from other lifetimes (e.g. a person has a phobic response in crowds and remembers a past-life of being killed when being mobbed).
c. <u>Emotional</u> residues exist from emotions that have been carried over from other life times. These emotions generally show up when triggered by specific topics or experiences (e.g. a client has no explanation for hatred or anger toward specific people, until she is regressed into a past-life and finds the same souls, in a past incarnation, who have betrayed her).

Past-life Therapy Techniques

Some of the same regression methods that were discussed in the previous chapter can be used in past-life therapy. These include differentiation, and desensitization. There are also other advanced past-life therapy techniques that may worth considering, such as the following:

1) Soul group recognition:

Many people believe that they have reincarnated with the same people in this life that they knew in previous lives. During past-life regressions, many experience powerful revelations when they are told to look into the eyes of a significant character within the memory. Christ said that "the eyes are the windows of the soul." Perhaps this is the reason that this form of recognition frequently occurs in these abstract regressions.

2) Transition Stage:

The death stage is one of the most important times to access for the purpose of therapy. At that moment, many of the residues that supposedly govern karma are prevalent. Thoughts, feelings, and other concepts, such as learning lessons, and that which was lost or gained, may be discussed and prove to be highly therapeutic. In addition, death is a very dramatic part of life which holds many mysteries to man's existence, so these experiences can be an important part of a client's hypnotherapy relative to his or her faith in the journey of the soul.

If a client had not yet encountered transition spontaneously during the regression, I will suggest that a client "go to the last day of (your) life" at the end of a past-life regression. This area holds a lot of information for the client.

3) Review Stage:

Often, individuals have found themselves floating up into a bright light after transition, where they are met by angels or spirit guides. In the light, often discovered is a review stage. If this is not found right away, we can suggest that the client find a place in the light where he or she can review the past-lifetime. This is where learnings are often discussed in more detail, sometimes with angelic or spiritual entities, and sometimes alone we might say.

The presence of "the light" that is described by some people at the end of a past-life regression is the same awesome, permeating feeling of unconditional love, wholeness, and peace as those who have had a near death experience report.

Two common results of past-life therapy

1) <u>Catharsis-</u> The client undergoes an abreaction and purifies emotional states. He or she experiences dissolution of unconscious "triggers" of various patterns in the present environmental conditions and circumstances in various relationships. There is an overwhelming sense of release of suppressed emotion and an unwinding of mental complexes.

2) <u>Symbolic Resonance Awareness-</u> The client begins to experience a deeper, inner understanding of the purpose for involvement in past and present relationships and situations. This leads to a mystical-spiritual integration of past memories and present-life circumstances. A greater sense of purpose is encountered relative to the divine and synchronistic aspects of destiny.

<u>Past-life Exploration:</u>

This process is similar to past-life therapy, except that there is no therapeutic goal. In this case, we may suggest that the client go back to "a past-life that is most important for (you) to remember at this time." Many people will often still experience catharsis during these memory experiences, which makes them therapeutic from time to time. A benefit is that sometimes this approach is less threatening for the client if the goal is just self-exploration, which is often the case when a person from the general public sets up an appointment specifically for past-life regression.

Transformational Models

Some of the best transformational models that I have used to help people transform problems by way of abstract regression include three models discussed in the previous chapter: differentiation, spirit guidance, and desensitization. I have recreated these to suit past-life memories as follows:

When a client seems to recall a past-life, at the end of the lifetime, I like to use what I call, "the mountain of time." There I ask the client to imagine both lifetimes, the past and the present. I ask what is similar and what is different, pointing out the patterns and learnings. Another effective tool, is to regress the client to pick up a spirit guide from either before birth, or have them meditate on "the light," where this is also accomplished. With the leadership of the client's guardian angel, or higher-self, the client is shown the most beneficial past-life. Another good model involves desensitization. When an emotionally loaded event is uncovered in an abstract regression, the memory segment is repeated several times by directing the client to, "Go back to the beginning of this memory and tell me the story again."

Past-life Research

It is not necessary to conduct research-oriented past-life regressions, unless the client has entered into hypnotherapy sessions with that specific purpose in mind. In this case, once the memory becomes vivid, the client may be asked research-oriented questions which pinpoint names, dates, and places. However, students of hypnotherapy should be cautioned that this may stir the logical mind, or the conscious mind, lightening the client's trance level. If this occurs, deepening the trance after asking such questions may be necessary. Popular tools used in research, with the goal of avoiding activating the conscious mind, include asking the client to find a local newspaper in the past-life and read the front page. This way the subconscious mind stays in an impressionistic mode, rather than being forced to rationalize the images. Another method is using words that indicate guessing, so that the client does not feel like he or she needs to be rationalize as much to be accurate, but just trust their impressions (e.g. "about how old are you?" or "What year comes to your mind?").

Research into these memories has often proved to be fruitful. Numerous books have been written exemplifying cases where hypnotically induced memories have been successfully documented in historical archives. In some cases, clients have found relatives they had left behind in a past-life, only to be reunited in the present. However, it is important to note that the majority of clients that enter into a hypnotherapist's office are geared toward specifically receiving the therapeutic value of the sessions, and are not interested in the research aspects of the work.

Some hypnotherapists automatically ask for this information, just in case the client requests such at the end of the session, while other hypnotherapists are more interested in clients' abilities to transform their limitations, experience the healing of their problems, and increase their awareness. Nonetheless, in several cases where my clients and I have embarked upon the purpose of obtaining verifiable information, and then later when we traced these paths through time, the results have been quite gratifying.

So the key to being a good regression therapist is to keep an open mind, remaining client-centered, while working with whatever information the client is bringing forward in the session. If the client wishes to validate memories or images later, this research approach should be established at the beginning of the session; if the memories and images simply prove to be therapeutic and healing, then this is just as productive, perhaps even more so when considering the resolution of karma, the enhancement of personal growth, and the expanded awareness gained from witnessing the journey of the soul.

Chapter 19

The Cayce Effect

A Brief History of Edgar Cayce

Because of his ability to enter into a state of self-hypnosis to diagnose illnesses and predict the future, Edgar Cayce was coined the "Sleeping Prophet." His talent first came to him when he was a 10 year old boy. Because he read the western biblical text once a year from cover to cover, an angel appeared to him and told him that because he was loyal to God, he would be granted a wish. When asked what he wanted, he replied, "I want to help people."

Thereafter, a series of events took place that led him to have a range of experiences that included osmosis, telepathy, the ability to read ailments in the body, and future prophecy. When he was a young man, he lost his voice. Upon encountering this problem, a hypnotist came into town to try to help him recover his speech. This was unsuccessful, by itself; but when he was hypnotized a second time, he gave himself a reading, and achieved success. Using the suggestions from the superconscious realm, he restored the circulatory functions of his vocal cords, and he was cured.

Although this set up a string of valuable healings that resulted from the readings, of which the media caught wind, he was not always in conscious agreement with the information that came through them. Some of the information which came through his readings, such as reincarnation, was not consistent with his more traditional Christian beliefs. Nonetheless, the popular "life readings," where he would read several of his client's past lives, became a popular aspect of his work. The uncanny accuracy of his health readings for those that were ill brought the attention of investors and resulted in the materialization of the Cayce Hospital, which was predicted in the readings and built in Virginia Beach, Virginia, in the early twentieth century.

Cayce passed away in 1945, but the Association for Research and Enlightenment (A.R.E.) maintains the 14000+ readings that still exist today for the benefit of the public in the A.R.E. library, one of several buildings that overlooks the Atlantic Ocean. This library carries the reputation of being the largest metaphysical and alternative medicine library in the world.

Many Cayce researchers claim that his prophecies have turned out to be quite accurate, such as his predictions of the great depression and World War II; and many claim that he accurately predicted significant events that are occurring in the present day. The wealth of information contained in the Edgar Cayce readings can be accessed for a variety of reasons, but for our purposes, I have decided to emphasize those concepts within the Cayce readings that are more closely related to transpersonal hypnosis.

Cayce's Categories of Mind Defined:

Edgar Cayce often utilized the collective unconscious, or the superconscious mind, to access information. Yet, in order to gain perspective on the Cayce categories of mind, we should look at the following Cayce descriptions and definitions of mind that came through his readings[14]:

3744.2 (Q3) "Definition of the word MIND."
(A) "That which is the active force in an animate object. ...Mind being that control of, or being the spark of the Maker, the WILL, the individual when we reach the plane of man. ...MIND is THAT that reasons the impressions from the senses, as they mani-

fest before the individual. ...The mind may be classified into the two forces: that between the physical and soul, and that between the soul and spirit force."

"Definition of the words CONSCIOUS MIND:"
"The CONSCIOUS means THAT that is able to be manifested in the physical plane through one of the senses."

"Definition of the word sub-conscious mind:"
"That lying between the soul and spirit forces within the entity, and is reached more thoroughly when the conscious mind is under subjugation of the soul forces of the individual or physical body. We may see (this) manifestation in those of the so-called spiritual minded people. The manifestation of the subconscious in their action. That portion of the body, better known as the one that propagates or takes care of the body—physical, mental, moral or what not, when it is not able to take care of itself."

"Subconscious is Unconscious force: This may be seen in every nerve end, in every muscular force. Subconscious action may be brought into manifestation by the continual doing of certain acts in the physical plane, so the body becomes unconscious of doing the acts that it does. ...Urges- Either astrological influences, resulting from experiences in planes of consciousness other than earth, or influences from the effects of retardment or advancement in previous lives on the earth."

900.31 (Q4) "Is it correct for (person 900) to say in his book that the superconscious is the mind or supreme controlling force of the Universal Forces?"

(A) "As pertaining to an individual, yes. As pertaining to Universal Forces, in the larger sense, no, but through the superconscious the Universal Forces are made active in subconsciousness. As is illustrated in the work as done through body, Edgar Cayce: through consciousness, the suggestion to the subconscious forces appertain to those conditions of the superconscious of the individual, coming then in touch with the Universal Forces in that manner and channel, for as the spiritual entity in its development has been in and partaken of the Universal forces in its development, the entity, when submerged from physical to that of superconscious and subconscious, appertain to those elements, and of that element the superconsciousness a portion of the great Universal Forces."

The Cayce Effect

Cayce described how he performed his readings in a few different ways, which can be documented in the readings themselves. When he entered into a state of self-hypnosis, he would often report a flash of light, which appeared to be the doorway for accessing various information. In some readings, Edgar Cayce described his encounter with "funnels," "spirals," or "cones," or what I refer to as "funnels of consciousness."

Each funnel of consciousness for each "entity," or human being, contains the four levels of mind, discussed previously as our basis for the mind process model. The conscious mind is the physical protrusion from the spirit realm into the material or physical plane of existence, which is symbolized as the tip of the funnel in the illustration that follows.

I perceive the *Cayce Effect* as the ability to enter into an altered state of consciousness and thereby transcend normal consciousness and the physical body—the most concrete part of mind, according to Cayce, up through the subconscious, unconscious, and superconscious levels of mind at the top. It is the top of the funnel that openly expands and connects to a vast amount of information, spiritual experiences, and to the creator. It is through the superconscious pathways that we human beings are connected to each other.

To better understand what I refer to as the Cayce Effect, let's assume that Edgar Cayce was one of the funnels of consciousness that touched down into the physical-material plane. In my opinion, when Cayce went into a self hypnotic state, his consciousness traveled up his funnel through the subconscious mind, through the unconscious mind, and into the superconscious realm. From there, his consciousness located another funnel of consciousness (another human being) and was able to read his client's uncon-

Cayce Effect Illustation

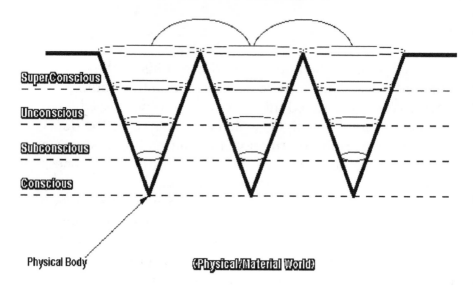

scious mind (past lives, tendencies, urges, etc.) their subconscious mind (current emotions and thoughts), and their conscious mind (decisions and physical health). It was then, when he reached the conscious level of an entity that he said, "We have the body" and gave the appropriate reading. In addition, he was able to do his most popular "Life Readings," where he allowed his consciousness to travel through the superconscious to a place called the akashic records. It was there that he read his client's past, present and future probabilities.

How accurate was Edgar Cayce? He is known by many metaphysicians and parapsychologists as the most accurate psychic of our time. Over time, researchers have been known to give Mr. Cayce an 85% accuracy rating. In the beginning days of giving readings, it was through his ability to access these areas of mind that Cayce astounded medical doctors. Before x-ray, some medical doctors relied on the readings for that purpose. Some physicians used Cayce's talents to further diagnose illness, and some used it for clarity on treatment plans. Most treatment plans which he recommended involved natural remedies, and some recommended surgery. Interestingly, one reading revealed that there was a natural cure somewhere on the planet for every ailment.

One of the first and most popular readings that resulted in a well documented cure was when Hugh Lynn Cayce, Edgar Cayce's son, burned his eyes with flash powder while playing in the family owned photography business. Edgar was told by medical doctors that his son would be permanently blind and in order to save his life, doctors recommended removing one eye. Instead of surgery, Hugh Lynn pleaded with his father to use the gift that God bestowed upon him, and with skepticism from the medical community, he agreed. Upon entering a state of self-hypnosis, in which he was very familiar, he was told to repetitively apply tannic acid on the boys eyes while in a dark room over a 15 day period. The bandages were peeled away and it was applied as stipulated in the reading. By the end of the specified period of time, the boy's eyes were miraculously healed.

Another well documented account of the impressive accuracy of the readings involves a woman going to Edgar Cayce for a health reading in Virginia Beach, at which time she was told to go to a specific local pharmacy in her home area of Kentucky where she was to ask for a remedy called "Oil of Smoke." She did as directed, but the pharmacist replied that he didn't carry it anymore. She contacted Edgar Cayce to report the unsuccessful result, so he went into trance again for more information. Shortly thereafter, he told her that she should go back to the pharmacist and ask him to look on the back row of a shelf in the back of the pharmacy. Indeed, it was there. The pharmacist was very surprised, because it had been on the back shelf for years, without his knowing.

This again demonstrates the accuracy of the Cayce readings. When he tapped into a funnel of consciousness of another "entity," as he referred, which could be somebody thousands of miles away, he discovered many details about a person who he had very little or no prior knowledge of beforehand.

Mr. Cayce was a Sunday school teacher for a Disciples of

Christ Christian church, so when his readings shifted from health readings to include past lives, he was very surprised. His own belief system did not at first embrace reincarnation. However, those that received the Life Readings, which often included this concept, were very contented to make sense of their soul's repetitive path through the earth plane, their present purposes in current-life relationships and situations, and their probable futures.

Incredibly, I met a few of those that Cayce read for who were still alive today and claimed their futures were read with 100% accuracy, including Edgar's grandson, Charles Thomas Cayce, whose reading was given to him when he was a young boy. Later in life, he found the reading written down on a sheet of paper, which confirmed everything had come true as predicted regarding his career choices, his future involvement with the A.R.E., and more.

How deep did Edgar Cayce go into a state of hypnosis? Objectively speaking, nobody knows exactly how deep Cayce went into the altered state, because the electroencephalogram was not invented at that time in order to be able to measure. However, by examining the chapter on depth correlations, we know that there is a positive correlation between depth and amnesia; a woman by the name of Gladys Davis recorded most of the readings because he went so deep that he became amnesiac (forgot what he had said) upon awakening. Based on this information, we know that Edgar Cayce must have gone into somnambulism and perhaps experienced delta brain waves, as some well-practiced yogis have been documented to achieve.

One interesting phenomenon, which may indicate the uniqueness of the altered state that Cayce achieved, was that of staying under hypnosis for an approximate 24 hour period of time. This occurred when somebody waved a piece of paper over Cayce's head. Perhaps the reason why he didn't awaken after that is because there was a part of his essence that actually left his body to travel into other dimensional realities, and when the paper was passed above his head, it broke the little silver cord. This is the cord that connects a person's soul awareness to their body, reported by many people who have had out-of-body or near-death experiences.

I believe it would be accurate for us to assume that Edgar

Cayce experienced deeper levels of self-hypnosis in a way that surpasses the vast majority of peoples' abilities in using self-hypnosis today.

Reproducing the Cayce Effect:

There are a few places in the files of the readings where Cayce described the objective (body preparation, etc.) and the subjective (mental imagery, etc.) processes by which his readings took place. As far as I am aware, there are only two hypnotic researchers that have been able to consistently reproduce the Cayce Effect, as I refer, and document it— Henry Leo Bolduc and Delores Cannon.

Ms. Cannon put somebody under hypnosis to reinterpret the life and prophecies of Nostradamus and Jesus Christ, but she did not share the process by which she hypnotized her subjects in her books. Bolduc, however, took information directly from the Cayce readings and specifically documented the process. In his book, *The Journey Within: Past Life Regression and Channeling,* he sets out to use hypnosis and the Cayce readings with specific individuals who are in turn able to reproduce the Cayce Effect while under a deep hetero-hypnotic trance.

Bolduc accesses Edgar Cayce Reading 294-19, which specifically describes how Cayce entered into and read the akashic records. He then takes the reading and transforms it into a script that he uses with his most susceptible subjects. He reads this script to these deeply hypnotized subjects and they begin to experience metaphysical phenomena that is very similar to that which Edgar Cayce encountered. Through the use of hypnosis, and utilizing the imagery process that which Edgar Cayce experienced, they effectively read the conditions of the mind and body in others, channel spirit guides, and read the akashic records.

The Collective Unconscious and Hypnotic Transference

If we were to examine the Cayce Effect Illustration and note that each person, represented by an individual funnel of consciousness, has his or her consciousness connected together by the superconscious mind, we could speculate that human beings share thoughts, particularly when in a state of hypnosis. In my opinion, the "collective unconscious," which Carl Jung referred to, is the same area that Edgar Cayce referred to as the akashic records.

The Cayce Effect is sometimes reproduced spontaneously in normal everyday clinical hypnotherapy sessions between the client and hypnotherapist. This occurs when a client's memory surfaces in the hypnotherapist's mind just before the client imagines it. In other words, the hypnotherapist recognizes that his or her own imagery may be reflecting the client's memories under regression, and then a short moment later this imagery is documented as being accurate when the client describes the same content in his or her own memory imagery. The hypnotherapist is receiving a psychic impression of sorts.

This mind-sharing effect occurs because every human being is connected to the superconscious realm, and the effect is amplified with hypnosis. It may be safe to assume that hypnosis makes people more intuitive. When a hypnotherapist puts an individual under hypnosis, this thought-sharing effect may occur because the hypnotherapist is inadvertently also putting him or herself under hypnosis at the same time. This is because the hypnotherapist is unconsciously listening to the same suggestions that he or she is describing to the client to induce hypnosis; and these are the same suggestions that were originally selected by the hypnotherapist, because he or she believed them to be effective on him or herself, and therefore on everyone else.

In general, the level achieved on ourselves by reading hypnotic induction scripts to others is a lighter level than that experienced by a hypnotherapy client, because of the conscious activity required of the practitioner in conducting the session. Yet, regardless of the trance level, hypnotherapists often can receive images that the client is experiencing before the client mentions them. Through long term private practice with hypnotic regression, this effect occurs more often; and as a result, hypnotherapists eventually become highly intuitive about others, even during their everyday lives.

Conversely, when the flow of information goes from hypnotherapist to client, because the client's sessions have opened them up to the collective unconscious, the effect is known as "hypnotic transference." In other words, clients may begin to receive the thoughts of their hypnotherapist. Generally, the more hypnosis sessions a client has, the more likely that this effect could take place. In essence, the client is clearing a path through the various levels of mind with each trance he or she experiences, which is progressively deeper and more permeating. As a result, the client travels through the three lower levels of mind and eventually reaches the superconscious realm of mind. This is why self-clearing exercises, which are discussed in the chapter on self-hypnosis, are important for hypnotherapists to do to maximize their effectiveness. It is important to be clear of issues, or problems, before entering into sessions with clients, in order to reduce hypnotic transference. When pondering the proper mind set of an effective therapist, consider what Carl Jung once said, "It's not what you say, it's who you are." After all, isn't intention really the key to a hypnotherapist's results? And intention can only come from within.

In one of his later books, *Memories, Dreams, Reflections*, Dr. Jung says, "The collective unconscious is common to all; it is the foundation of what the ancients called 'sympathy of all things'."[15] He goes on to describe two instances of a similar effect to hypnotic transference, which I refer to as collective unconscious transfer. In both cases, Carl Jung experienced the world of his clients by receiving physical and mental manifestations within himself that existed simultaneously in his clients. In one case, Jung had a precognitive dream about a lady. Shortly thereafter, he recognized a woman in his office as the lady in his dream. Later, another dream involving the same client occurred between sessions, and in the next session, he was able to perceive her religious conflicts more accurately and then effectively help her solve her problems. In another case a client died from a gunshot wound to the head, and at the same time Dr. Jung received a pain in the same area of his own head. Because of his awareness level, he knew that the collective unconscious was giving him an accurate impression regarding his client.

To summarize the information in this chapter, we must take into consideration the function of the four primary levels of the mind. The superconscious mind is an important area of consideration in transpersonal hypnotherapy, because without a good connection to it, the client is cut off from receiving spiritual information which may be helpful in guiding his or her life. If it is part of the client's goal, the superconscious may be used to access spirit guides, or between life/after life memories, and more. Yet, most problems that hypnotherapists encounter seem to exist in the client's unconscious mind. This is the place where a person's past programming seems to be holding him or her back in some way; and hypnotherapy is the only bridge that can be utilized to effectively change these unconsciously rooted problems.

All four levels of mind interact and have permeable boundaries, in order to cocreate our awareness. They all function synchronistically with each other increasing the other's effectiveness. As a result, there is only a subtle difference between these levels for people who practice altered states of consciousness. However, for those who do not, there is a limited understanding of the distinction between each level of mind, and the experiences each level has to offer relative to hypnotic phenomena.

More Resources on this Chapter

There is more information that refers to the readings of Edgar Cayce throughout this book; however, natural limitations exist when considering the vast amount of information contained in the library of readings available at the Association for Research and Enlightenment (A.R.E.). For further information, contact the A.R.E. or read, *There is a River,* by Thomas Sugrue. Another fabulous piece of work that further explains the inner-workings of the mind's intuitive process is a book titled, *The Intuitive Heart,* by Henry Reed, Ph.D..

In a transpersonal context, and throughout the Cayce readings, a common theme is that the mind, body, and spirit affect each other, and hypnosis is "the bridge" for crossing these three dimensions of human existence.

Cayce Reading 349.4 - "For the spirit is the life; the mind is the builder; the physical is the result."

Chapter 20

Dangers and Precautions

There are guidelines I will share that most hypnotherapists generally use to operate a private practice. I have never seen anybody harmed by hypnosis in well over two decades teaching hypnotherapy and conducting private practice with literally thousands of people. Nonetheless, it is good to have a practical notion of how to practice hypnotherapy with the highest regard for the client. A historical piece of advice from the medical profession in the United States for medical doctors is, "Physician Do No Harm." When reading this chapter, it is important to note that I am a self-pronounced humanitarian and not a legal authority. It is also important to keep in mind that there are literally thousands of different self-hypnosis tapes for sale to the general public, from which many people have benefited safely for decades.

All hypnosis is self-hypnosis, since it occurs within the individual and is not an external event. In other words, individuals don't actually get put under hypnosis, they simply agree to imagine the things that they are experiencing. A suggestion is just that, a *suggestion*, not a *command*. There is an internal-subconscious stage of agreement to imagine and experience suggestions. *Everything* is a suggestion and it is up to each individual to agree or disagree to experience it. In general, the more a person focuses on suggestions, the more real those ideas become. Under hypnosis, suggestions are imagined more vividly, however, there is still an agreement to accept the suggestion to the point of actually experiencing it. In addition, hypnotherapy clients suggest much to themselves while in trance, particularly when giving reality to their memory images in a regression.

I remember one psychologist who graduated from my course and made up a disclaimer that said something to the effect, "I agree fully to put myself under hypnosis with the suggestions that I am given, and I take full responsibility for whatever comes to my mind. I am responsible for determining whether or not it is real or unreal, and what I should do with the information. I will hold harmless..."

I am not sure we need to go this far to achieve the goal of self preservation, but there are many ways to do so if we feel it is necessary. Hypnotherapists may consider liability insurance through National Association of Transpersonal Hypnotherapists listed in the Afterword. Some intake forms ask if the client has ever sued anybody before, to detect a pattern. In addition, practicing prayer, faith, and a higher intention is a great, natural insurance policy to take into account. Each individual may want to consider this concept when regularly practicing.

This, of course, could lead to many discussions regarding politics and philosophy, which has to do with individual choice, so we will avoid going further into this direction and continue to talk about what *rarely* but could go wrong, and the precautions we can take to exercise prevention.

As readers examine what follows, it is important to remember that individuals are resilient, and they normalize quickly and easily.

Dangers and Precautions

1) Neglect of Suggestion Removal:
a) Hallucination- This problem can occur with entertainment hypnosis. When an individual is given a suggestion to imagine something that doesn't exist in the material world as suggested, a hallucination occurs. In some cases, for entertainment purposes, a

subject is given a humorous suggestion, such as butterflies flying in front of his or her face when he or she hears somebody cough. If this suggestion is not removed after the demonstration, he or she could randomly hear a cough and then see a brief image of butterflies in front of his or her eyes, causing visual disruptions or distortions and leading to an accident, although I have never heard of this occurring. Fortunately, as with all cases of hypnosis, homeostasis—a natural state of balance, will soon occur even without suggestion removal.

Precaution: When doing entertainment hypnosis, just before awakening the subject, tell him or her that all of the suggestions given are canceled and everything is back to normal.

b) *Amnesia*- This problem also can occur with entertainment hypnosis. If an individual is told to forget the number seven, and the suggestion is not removed, he or she may have difficulty adding or multiplying with sevens. This would be difficult only for a short period of time (minutes or hours); nonetheless, it could cause a problem until homeostasis takes place.

Precaution: Just before awakening, tell the client that all the suggestions given are canceled and everything is back to normal. Normalization often occurs by itself anyway, since illogical suggestions don't last very long after hypnosis, in the event that they are not removed.

2) Ill-timed Anesthesia:

This problem can occur with posthypnotic suggestions only. Hypothetically speaking, a client is told that a part of the body will go numb when a specific stimulus occurs, such as a snap of the fingers. Thereafter, when the client hears someone snap his or her fingers, a numbness may be experienced without the client consciously consenting to it at that time.

Precaution: It is recommended that the hypnotherapist not use a common stimulus as a post hypnotic key, such as the snap of the fingers. Instead, if the hypnotherapist uses a hypnoanesthetic key, he or she should use a wrist pull. It is very rare that this key is unintentionally triggered and random numbness occurs. In addition, the numbing effect very rarely occurs without the client also sitting in a relaxing chair in a quiet area. As a result, the snap sound may be ignored by the subconscious mind, even if the suggestion were not removed.

3) Suggestion Denial Produces Anxiety:

The easiest and most comfortable condition for the client is the scenario where the client is following the majority of the suggestions that he or she has been given, thus engaging in new habits that were hypnotically suggested. If the client is denying a large majority of the suggestions, he or she may have an internal battle occurring in the mind, or a conflict of motivations. When inner motivational conflict peaks, some clients may experience a higher amount of anxiety than usual. This can be the case for those attempting to change a longtime habit. There is a feeling of wanting to engage in the old habit and, at the same time, subconscious hypnotic suggestions are urging the client to engage in new habits or behaviors.

Precaution: What I have done in the past with middle-of-the-road clients is to ask them at the second session, when anxiety is evident, to get off of the fence. In other words, the client is encouraged to make the conscious decision of which direction he or she would like to go... stay with the old habits or commit to the new ones. If the client still wants to change, a good interview is necessary in order to change past programming, or associations, and create suggestions that are more appealing toward the desired change. Sometimes, stern encouragement may be necessary, so that clients in this predicament will make the best conscious decisions for themselves during times of challenge.

4) Ignorance of Physical Problems:

There are a myriad of physical ailments which would be helpful for a hypnotherapist to become aware of. A person could have a heart problem and an abreaction under hypnotic regression could make it worse. An individual could have diabetes, and weight loss suggestions could cause further health problems. In addition, although medical hypnosis research shows hypnosis reduces epileptic seizures, an epileptic person, hypothetically, could have a seizure sometime during a session and we may simply write it off as a useful catharsis. Another problematic client may be the psychiatric patient who is seeking hypnotherapy for medicated conditions, such as schizophrenia or hallucination. This client-type is generally not a candidate for hypnotherapy.

Precautions: A good personal history is helpful, most of which could be included on the confidential interview form furnished by most hypnotherapy training institutes. These forms ask clients to list heart problems, diabetes, epilepsy, and other physical or psychological conditions, and the contact information of their medical and mental health providers, with a request for permission to contact them. Some health problems require a written referral from a physician, in order for a hypnotherapist to work with them, depending on local laws—which often vary.

Most hypnotherapists work with the normal and functional person in everyday society. This client-type generally keeps the certified hypnotherapist very busy, even without any other licenses in other practices. I tend to practice by the motto, "When in doubt, do without, or give the physician a shout." A hypnotherapist's client load generally consists of smoking, weight loss, and various stress conditions. Therefore, the client with a multiplicity of problems can be referred to choose from a few mental health or medical professionals in the local community. Hypnotherapy is effective for people who have a goal orientation, or an idea of what they need to work on. Hypnotherapy clients need the ability to focus on one goal at a time, both in the normal waking state and while under hypnosis.

5) Using hypnoanesthesia without prior medical research into the cause of the pain:

Pain is a signal that the body uses for self preservation. It exists for us to be able to recognize that something is wrong with the body that requires our attention. If hypnosis, or other anesthetic treatments, remove pain before determining its cause, there is a danger that the body's needs are being neglected and therefore further injury is possible.

Precaution: In order to ensure safe hypnoanesthesia, it is best to get a letter from a medical doctor indicating hypnoanesthesia would be beneficial to a particular patient. Also, through the client interview forms discussed earlier, a hypnotherapist may have permission to contact the client's physician and obtain the needed information.

Sometimes, the body has its own agenda regardless of the use of hypnoanesthesia. For example, I remember a psychologist who took my training program and then successfully underwent a root canal using self-hypnosis exclusively as the anesthetic agent. During her post surgery recovery, she called the institute's offices concerned that the self-hypnosis she was using on her tooth pain wasn't effective anymore, because she was very uncomfortable. I explained that the body may be communicating to her that there was something wrong, which is probably why it wasn't giving her as much numbness as before. Sure enough, when she went back to the dentist to get the root canal checked, he found an abscess that needed medical attention. She was amazed at the body's ability to communicate.

In summary, it is best to obtain written permission from a client's medical doctor, before using hypnoanesthesia. However, the mind and body have an integral relationship that is part of homeostasis that makes the use of hypnoanesthesia fairly safe. The human mind has a relationship with the body whereby it generally allows or disallows hypnoanesthesia on the long term.

6) Ignorance of the Audience:

Suggestion has full power to an observer, or an audience in the case of group hypnosis or stage hypnosis. This may cause an unintentional and unattended abreaction. Whether it is a spouse that came into the room to observe a session, or it is one person out of 25 that came to a group hypnosis workshop, these people may need individual attention if or when a negative memory or experience arises while they are under hypnosis. If it happens in a group, it is often inconvenient for the hypnotherapist to tend to just one person. In entertainment hypnosis, some observers go under hypnosis, just by simply watching the process that is occurring on stage.

Precaution: In entertainment hypnosis, the stage hypnotist can ask the audience, "Whoever is under hypnosis in the audience, please raise your hand. You are no longer under hypnosis; you're wide awake now if you are in the audience." In group hypnosis, if it is inconvenient for the hypnotherapist to handle the problem at that time, he or she may go to the unattended observer, who is under hypnosis and abreacting, and suggest that whatever he or she is experiencing at the time is "fading away like a dream" and that he or she will work on it later. Then, it is usually best to refocus the individual onto some pleasant imagery. In group hypnotic regressions, a hypnotherapist may utilize a "spotter." This is generally a hypnotherapist who spots and handles abreactions in the audience, while the leading hypnotherapist, who is guiding the group, continues with the group hypnosis process.

7) Hypnotherapy may uncover an amnesiac trauma:

On rare occasion, a hypnotherapist and his or her client may become surprised at what the subconscious mind brings to light. Sometimes negative memories from the past surface spontaneously when and if the client's subconscious mind desires resolution. However, most of the time, these unpleasant images surface as a result of hypnotic regression, and it is not a surprise, due to the fact that both parties discussed the potential of such memories surfacing beforehand.

The fact that these may surface does not pose a problem by itself; however, one of the most frequent mistakes made by beginning hypnotherapists involves awakening a client while he or she is in the middle of an abreaction. In these cases, the client may be mentally reviewing the things that he or she remembered and suggested to themselves while under hypnosis for the next several hours, or perhaps even days. The client's subconscious mind will perform stress rehearsal, or repetitively rerun the memory, until the feeling or memory has been resolved. Sometimes therapists awaken a client out of an abreaction, because the client's session is running over into another client's scheduled session time. This scenario, if possible, should be avoided.

Precaution: It is best to wait until the memory has run its course to a point of temporary resolution, if possible. Once a sense of tiredness or peacefulness occurs, as is observed in the client, it may be assumed that the memory segment has at least been temporarily resolved. Thereafter, perhaps during the post session interview, a hypnotherapist may want to consider whether or not he or she desires to handle the emotional magnitude that is likely to occur in future sessions with that specific client. If not, a mental health practitioner who has experience with highly abreactive clients can use more conscious-mind oriented therapies, which can give clients a better understanding of themselves and their conditions.

Some hypnotherapists feel a calling to work with clients with post traumatic stress memories and the resulting cathartic hypnotherapy sessions. Because one session of hypnosis is equal to ten sessions of psychotherapy, it is often best for counseling or psychotherapy clients to have access to hypnotherapy at some point in their path of recovery. If a mental health professional is not thoroughly trained in hypnotherapy, this can be accomplished by splitting sessions between a hypnotherapist and a licensed mental health professional.

For example, Lynne D. Finney MS, JD, author of *Reach For The Rainbow*, stated that her recovery from sexual abuse was first facilitated through a hypnotherapist. Shortly thereafter, she learned self-hypnosis and began regressing herself into her own forgotten traumatic memories, and then later engaged in counseling for finishing her recovery. I say, "To each his own," when clients choose their practitioners and methods for their path of healing; so it is good to help clients look at all the therapy modalities that are available to them when they have bigger goals in mind for themselves.

Considering Precautions and Dangers

Transpersonally speaking, if the student of hypnotherapy acts out of the highest intention, those intentions will manifest in positive ways. Spiritual relationship is the key to faith; and having the faith that the highest good for client and therapist will prevail is a must to be effective and maintain a sense of peace within a service profession.

The worst thing I've ever seen occur in my private practice is when an individual falls emotionally out of sorts for several hours, or perhaps days, due to an intense regression. It's a rare occurrence, but feeling out of balance can happen for some clients. In these cases, usually a monumental healing is at the end of the suffering. Once they have gone through this stage, they reach a state of balance again, and much more so than where they started.

Thank God, literally, for *homeostasis*, the innate human ability to know right from wrong, pain from pleasure, and the ability to regain a sense of balance within mental, emotional, and physical states after experiencing adversity. Without homeostasis, there would be no gage of normalcy within each human being.

Essentially, what I am suggesting is that human beings are resilient. A difficult experience is easily rectified, in time, with a sum totaling of all of our life experiences, which includes the pleasurable ones as well. The vast majority of clients respond to the most difficult memories with simply healing old wounds. It all comes down to hypnotherapists trusting the process and clients trusting their ability to heal.

It is always amazing to hear stories about people who were confronted with life threatening situations and responded by saving someone's life. They responded unconsciously and almost automatically. When these heroes were asked how they did it, they often respond with, "I didn't think about it. I just did it." Sometimes hypnotherapists simply need to trust their innate abilities, and teach their clients to do the same.

Chapter 21

The Transpersonal Approach

The transpersonal approach may be likened to a reading performed by Edgar Cayce which indicated that spirit is the life, mind is the builder, and body is the result. If there is a physical problem, there is a higher purpose for having the illness that is generally spiritually driven. If there is a mental problem, perhaps there is a higher spiritual purpose for having the difficulty, and a physical result as well. If there is a spiritual problem, such as a lack of faith, or perhaps a disconnection from a higher power, then there are often problems on mental, emotional, or perhaps even physical levels. The transpersonal approach emphasizes that the body, mind, and spirit affect each other, and hypnosis is the primary catalyst to bridge the three. By observing and watching for this triad when it is integrally at work, a hypnotherapist may become more effective with his or her clients. This higher level of effectiveness may be accomplished with indirect suggestions during an interview, or within the ability to offer more transpersonal hypnotherapeutic interventions.

Sometimes, there are more difficult client cases where the answer to the problem may not be as easily recognized by hypnotherapist and/or client. However, because the unconscious mind holds all of the answers to the body-mind-spirit triad, the client will often be able to undergo hypnosis and tell a hypnotherapist details concerning the origin of his or her problem, and sometimes even how to resolve it.

By recognizing that each individual has a higher power that is present or accessible within his or her life in its own unique way, the transpersonal hypnotherapist may simply serve as a *facilitator*, thus avoiding the "Guru" effect, or creating followers. In transpersonal hypnotherapy, the client feels self empowered during therapy, which overflows into his or her everyday life. Therefore, there is a longer lasting effect to the therapeutic changes as well.

If a higher power is believed by both parties to be directing the session, then both hypnotherapist and client are able to make progress more quickly. Because the value systems allow for the perception that the higher power in life is "God" or "Spirit" and not the therapist, there is a reduced risk of fostered dependency. There are many ways to include a client's spiritual path in hypnotherapy sessions; these can be both overt and covert.

Covert inclusions are probably the most important because the hypnotherapist's mind set is the most important factor in the equation for success. These can be done through regular prayer and faith, and the development of the hypnotherapist's spiritual relationship with a higher power, which can often shed light on sessions. This light can empower the hypnotherapist to be a facilitator with greater inner strength, a strength which is necessary for clarity within sessions and achieving longevity in a career of transforming problems. The benefits of serving others in such a personal way then stays rewarding each day.

Overt inclusions are also important, since a client will generally respond better to anything— therapy, life, etc... with a sense of a higher power. Overt inclusions may involve simply asking clients what their concept is of a higher power. This is not done with an agenda. Instead, it is done with an understanding that there are many paths, and if the creator allows many paths for finding and connecting with him/her, then a therapist would be more effective working within that framework as well.

Sometimes I ask clients what their beliefs are, what religion they practice, and/or I will ask them how they make "the connection." The connection is what I am trying to discover with the client, because if I become the facilitator, I also want to trust that clients have helpers afterthey no longer have me as a regular part of their lives.

If I am just going to see a client for two suggestive therapy sessions for a habit, we are usually not involved with deeper structure involving core values. In other cases, when I discover that a client lacks the connection to a higher source, and because that client would be at a higher level of peace if he or she had one, we often brainstorm ways to enter into some experiential spiritual experiences using hypnosis. A similar effect could be obtained by getting a reading from an accurate psychic, joining a meditation group, or entering into a formal religion or some type of prayer experience. Whatever he or she is open to is fine by me. There are many ways to make the connection, and each individual is most comfortable doing it in his or her own unique way.

Transpersonal hypnotherapists generally withhold judgment. Each individual is on their own unique path through human life, thus, each plays a different part on the stage of life's synchronistic paths. Each individual has an internal gauge for knowing the difference between right and wrong, light from dark, or good from bad, so *judgment* therefore becomes only a reflection of the judger. Understanding, on the other hand, comes from taking a higher perspective. Often those higher perspectives, or big picture thinking, can help a hypnotherapist have faith that life is just and good in the long run. Pain and healing have positive intentions behind them for a greater role in the grand scheme of things.

Those who seek new understandings generally find them, and these individuals often lead others to do the same. Hypnotherapists are more effective by submitting themselves to hypnotherapeutic processes, as a client, on a semi-regular basis. As a result, they can teach clients from a perspective of *wisdom*—having experienced the change process, rather than a limited base of *knowledge*—having only studied therapeutic theories. This wisdom will always serve to empower hypnotherapists and their clients on a much deeper and greater level.

Client-Centered Hypnotherapy

~

"I never try to convert a patient to anything, and never exercise any compulsion. What matters most to me is that the patient should reach his own view of things."[16]

Carl Jung

~

If we were to take another look at the history of hypnosis, we would find that most methods were practiced with an *authoritarian methodology*, leading people to believe that this method was most effective. This was true even during Milton Erickson's era, where he would give many of his subjects a "doctor's order" in order to motivate them to follow suggestions. It wasn't until recently, from about 1980 on, that hypnosis was perceived as being most effective when utilized with more *permissive methods*.

The permissive approach revolves around client-centered hypnotherapy. Ironically, Erickson could also be included in this category as he brought his patients' issues out into the open rather quickly and effectively, because he established rapport early in his sessions, which enabled his clients to promptly share the depths of their problems with him. When considering the awesome power of the unconscious mind in its ability to reveal the source of a problem, Erickson had been known to say, "trust the unconscious." This process of trusting a client's unconscious information occurs both in the interview process, as well as while a client is under hypnosis.

This is so important; I cannot stress it enough. If the hypnotherapist encourages clients to trust themselves, and their own mental content, it results in more self-empowerment. There is no way any therapist could understand the complete scope of a client's problem, as well as the client understands it, by just spending one or two hours in a session. Therefore, it is the responsibility of the hypnotherapist to build rapport quickly, and effectively draw the client's problem out. Helping clients focus on their needs, find the answers to their problems, and then act upon the information we get during an interview or intervention are the keys to successful client-centered hypnotherapy.

One way to create a client-centered environment is to utilize a good client interview method that automatically makes the client feel understood, which is the key to building rapport. Other methods that are commonly utilized by hypnotherapists include non-directive techniques, which probe the unconscious mind to discover answers. Methods where the therapist performs functions that encourage a client to formulate answers to their problems either consciously—during an interview, or unconsciously—while under hypnosis, may be considered client-centered.

If we were to look at trusting the unconscious mind of our client for the answers from a more transpersonal level, we can include the spiritual pathways of our client. In some cases, the life path that the client has taken up to the point of therapy is astounding. It can be very different from our own. If we are to be effective, obtaining results often requires embracing the client's path and furthering them along it as best we can. Sometimes we see the pot of gold at the end of the rainbow, yet we only work on the next step, as the client perceptually sees it. The client is only aware of the ladder that reaches the first or second color in the spectrum. This is because that is where the client perceives themselves, and they may not hear anyone who talks about the gold. The path therefore should be honored, and the therapeutic goal set by the client embraced, in order to be most effective.

Any time we accept a new client into private practice, we are embracing the client's goal as being equally as important to us, the hypnotherapist, as it is to the client. *Goal centered hypnotherapy,* is a way of practicing hypnotherapy whereby the hypnotherapist accepts the client's goal and agrees to be hired, or paid, to utilize his or her tools to the best of his or her abilities in order to achieve the stated goal. The client chooses the goal, and the therapist conducts sessions that revolve around it.

In general, the hypnotherapist never changes the original goal the client was expecting to work on. The only exception, if we are to be goal centered in our approach, is if the client brings up a new goal during the session. Sometimes, the client recognizes that the session is flowing in a new direction and begins to request that the goal of therapy be changed in some way. However, the vast majority of the time, the momentum a client brings into a session never changes. He or she has usually spent hours or perhaps years thinking about his or her problem and how someone will assist their goal at some point in the future. I prefer to be the facilitator that lies somewhere within the client's perceptual reality to assist in reaching their goal.

One of the most common case histories I share with my students, which is an example of goal-centered hypnotherapy involves a woman who wanted to quit smoking to lift her depression. She told me that she divorced about 1 1/2 years ago and that since then, she had stayed home and smoked in the evening and weekends instead of socializing, or going out places. She said that she was very depressed. I remember questioning whether or not smoking cessation was really what she needed to work on, when she showed signs of depression and being in the stages of grief. Nonetheless, I remained committed to this one rule for determining therapeutic goals — *working within the clients belief system will generally result in the greatest chance for success.* Since she claimed that her depression and hibernation behavior would disappear when she quit smoking, I needed to be willing to act upon that belief to assist her goal. In addition, since clients know themselves much better than I could ever get to know them in a matter of one hour, I must trust their beliefs about themselves first before my own. As a result, she did indeed quit smoking, and after further contact in the following week, I found out that her depression was lifting and she had more energy, which led to her going out more and socializing, as she had predicted.

In some rare cases, however, the hypnotherapist may find a conflict between his or her beliefs and the client's beliefs. Therefore, there is a conflict in therapeutic goals. For example, an anorexia client that wants to lose weight. It obviously could be dangerous if a hypnotherapist were to represent such a goal. Therefore, in these cases, there is a beliefs and values conflict between hypnotherapist and client, and the client either agrees to change the goal, or pursues it somewhere else. In essence, the hypnotherapist either takes the case by embracing the belief structure and goal of the client, or he or she rejects it. Perhaps, in this case, the goal could be changed, if the client sees that the goal is irrational when the hypnotherapist confronts him or her.

In another case history I can share, the session went a different direction when a woman came in to quit smoking. After the first session, she smoked no cigarettes until she was socializing, at which time she started smoking a few cigarettes again. At the second session I asked her if she felt more relaxed using hypnosis to quit smoking, and she said, "Yes." I asked her if she felt like she really had to have a cigarette, and she said, "No." Then, I reiterated that the two benefits of using hypnotherapy to quit smoking (relaxation and attitude adjustment) had been accomplished, and so I asked her, "So why did you smoke?" She responded with tears welling up in her eyes, "Because I fail at everything."

I realized at that moment we were talking about an ineffective belief structure which disabled her from being successful with probably anything she tried, let alone addiction cessation. I asked, "When did you start believing that?" She said, "My father used to tell me that I was a failure as far back as I can remember." She was starting to express more emotion, as I began to recognize that the goal of therapy was shifting.

I immediately explained how hypnotic regression therapy, utilizing wounded child imagery, may help her change that belief, and then it would be easier for her to quit smoking, or succeed at anything she tried for that matter. She agreed to try it, closed her eyes again, and I used the affect bridge to bridge the emotion back to its source. We performed the wounded child transformational model within the memory she had. (Wounded Child Blending is explained briefly in the chapter on regression.)

This resulted in some wonderful life-transformative results, but it is important to remember that changing a goal midstream, we might say, is a last resort. In 99% of my cases, I stay with the original goal(s) that were listed at the beginning of the first session.

One Goal At A Time

A client may bring multiple goals into a hypnotherapy session; however, the most important goal should be selected with the agreement of working toward accomplishing just one goal at a time (e.g. a person wants to simultaneously quit smoking and lose weight). The less important goal can be worked on after the client has accomplished the first goal.

This is what distinguishes hypnotherapy from psychotherapy. If a client discusses several goals at length, perhaps to a point of confusion, he or she may be better off engaging in psychotherapy as opposed to, or in addition to, hypnotherapy. The ideal hypnotherapy client is goal oriented from the start. They know what they want to work on, and this clarity is what the hypnotherapist relies upon for choosing a hypnotherapeutic intervention. If a client has more than one goal, then it is better to list them separately and work on each of these approximately 30 days apart. This allows the client to concentrate on changing one thing at a time and will usually render the best results.

Once I entered into private practice, I had noticed that people who became therapy clients sometimes expected me to know them better than they knew themselves. As a result, I began to create ways to self empower my clients to trust their own answers about themselves, and life in general. After practicing for well over a decade now, I still come to the same conclusion, client-centered and goal oriented hypnotherapy is the most effective; and it is more ecological in the many various contexts of living life.

~

"Faith is the trust that, given the love and power of God, and the freedom of the soul to choose, my brother (or sister) is better off on the path they and God have chosen, than the one you would choose for them."

Search For God, Book I

~

Interpersonal Variables Of Private Practice

One of the most challenging things for a new hypnotherapist to do is begin engaging in the therapist's role and making it a new profession. Four primary experiences that I have had when I was just starting out in private practice helped me get through my first year, and they later became the primary principles of the transpersonal hypnotherapeutic approach that I continue to depend upon.

Five Primary Principles for
Practicing Transpersonal Hypnotherapy

1) <u>Higher-Self Principle:</u> The client's higher self, the part that is spiritually aware of its true nature and its relationship to the creator, the part that is aware of its link to the superconscious (higher powers), knows beforehand that the hypnotherapist has something that the client needs to learn. This higher self is aware that the new hypnotherapist is just starting out to practice on others, and it is willing to also teach the hypnotherapist something unique that the hypnotherapist must learn as well. Even though this exchange is not consciously revealed, there is an unconscious awareness that it exists. There is a willingness to enter into the divine enlightened state of hypnosis, in order to let this unique process unfold. Therefore, for some unknown yet higher spiritual purpose, client and hypnotherapist have come together in a divinely guided relationship to experience this process and learn from each other.

When I first started out in private practice, this gave me the confidence then, and still gives me the confidence now after all of these years, to be patient with myself and to receive training from my greatest teachers, my clients. It always amazes me that when I learn a new technique, a client shows up with the condition that demands its use. I've also noticed that at least one client in my case load always seems to bring to me a subject matter that I am personally working on within myself. However, this is never revealed, since I am there on a conscious level for the client. After submitting myself to thousands of hours of education and training,

I still believe that the client is the greatest teacher, which makes me a permanent student of trance therapies, as well as human life.

2) <u>Self Empowerment Principle:</u> I often felt responsible for the client's problem when I first started out, because I was and am empathic and compassionate. As a result, I almost couldn't shoulder my clients' burdens within the first year of practice. The concept that some people actually come to a therapist believing that they are *broken* and someone else, the therapist, is going to *fix* them perplexed me. It was in my first year of practice that I took a workshop involving spiritual approaches to hypnotherapy that I was warned, "People will give their power up to you." I didn't quite know what my teachers meant until later, when a few of my clients did exactly that. I was the guru, they were the followers. Thereafter, once I discovered that this concept was possible from time to time, because of the nature of the therapeutic relationship, I developed ways to change this relationship dynamic.

I found that the only way to true healing and transformation is to self empower the client. Many people believe that all hypnotherapists are authoritarian therapists, which can make this transition even more difficult in the hypnotherapeutic relationship. After all, on TV it appears that they command the client to do what they are told. If the brain washing effect worked, then the therapy must be successful, when in fact this is furthest from the truth.

The hypnotherapeutic relationship is simply a dance of rapport. If rapport exists, the client is open to suggestions. From there, if the client has sound logical reasons to accept those suggestions, long-term therapeutic results take place. Transpersonal hypnotherapists have the greatest ability to self empower clients with the client-centered approach.

The first principle in client-centered hypnotherapy is trust the unconscious; the client has all the answers. If they claim that they are ignorant to the cause of their problems, clients will soon come up with their own answers when the altered state of hypnosis is applied and they are asked to reveal them.

3) <u>Physician/Healer, Heal Thyself Principle:</u> This particular saying comes from Paul in the new testament of the western biblical

text where he says, "Physician, heal thyself." It reflects the need for
the healer to be able to heal themselves through their own methods
in order to be effective in healing others. When hypnotherapists experience their own unconscious process of transformation through
self-hypnosis or hypnotherapy (with another hypnotherapist), they
become more effective hypnotherapists themselves. My favorite
saying to my advanced student is, "When a hypnotherapist walks
the path of healing, he or she may take others by the hand and
show them the way."

Due to submitting myself to approximately 100 or more
sessions of hypnotherapy, over the years, I have come to a comfortable place within myself, which I have known to rely on for a
great sense of peace and strength. Most of my character building
types of sessions were done in the first year. However, from time
to time, I still benefit from having a hypnotherapy session. When
I choose a trance therapist, I choose someone who is not overly
directive (having an agenda outside of mine), and who allows
me to have and define my own experiences. The benefits I receive
range from various forms of stress relief, to obtaining deeper more
profound levels of transcendental or spirit-guide hypnomedita-
tions. It may be accurate to say that the second greatest teacher is
ourselves, when we are in the client role.

4) <u>I Am What I Learn Principle:</u> Teachers of therapists can
play the role of mentor, therapist, or trainer. Regardless if we
choose a minister to open ourselves up with, a therapist, or a
hypnotherapy trainer, it leaves us with the same effect. They have
captured a rare glimpse of our humanness, or facilitated our inner
selves' evolutionary process. This is a lasting impression. In addition, interventions learned in class are modeled by the student in
various ways in the future.

A medical intuit that was a student of mine once told me,
"I'm very selective with the people I train under, because I don't
want them to influence me and the way I do things, unless I am
sure it is coming from a higher place." It is wise to select trainers
with discernment, because all personal growth experiences effect
our internal being. As a result of taking a training, at least for the
next few months or more, we will use the newest models of therapy

we learned from the training. If these models are taught with a higher intent, then they will be ecological, or good for everybody on all levels.

The most valuable hypnotherapy trainers that I have studied under were more like servants. They had a humbleness. They facilitated my finding my needs within a group setting, and both consciously and unconsciously taught me about myself. They provided me with a foundation of models and case histories for an applicable meaning to my learning experiences.

During advanced training courses, if the hypnotherapy trainer is not willing to share how he or she used his or her advanced tools to successfully heal some of the more intense clients, he or she is not serving students in the ways that are optimal. I generally say at the beginning of my classes, "I don't have any answers, I can only share my knowledge and my experiences with you. It is up to each of you to find your own answers." Then, I proceed to tell stories of success, for the most part, but I also share stories of trials where I had to make some sound decisions regarding client types and goals.

I must add that the best therapists and trainers that I have experienced also have had a good sense of humor. It seemed that at the most important times, I was taught to laugh, not take myself or the human plight too seriously. Humor, in good taste, is healing.

5) <u>Relationship Definition Principle:</u> One of the most difficult concepts for new hypnotherapists is the concept of charging money for helping people; yet, without this form of energy exchange, it is impossible for a hypnotherapist to exist in the physical world. As a result, it is necessary to create, embrace, and follow certain philosophies for conducting a private practice.

In my first year of being a hypnotherapist, when I was just in my mid-twenties, I experienced stress over the false idea that people were paying me for results. I thought that when I obtained success with clients, I was worthy of being paid. When I didn't get results, I felt like a failure that was undeserving. In order to avoid the roller coaster ride of conducting a new private practice, it became important to find ways to sustain a position of internal strength, not only for my clients, but for myself. The stronger that I became within myself, the more effective I became as a therapist. In order to create more inner strength, I knew that I had to appropriately detach, while maintaining an adequate level of compassion, in order to be effective.

It wasn't long before I defined my role as a therapeutic landlord. I began to take on the perspective that I possessed certain properties, or hypnotherapy skills and tools, which people were renting. When they paid for a session, they were supporting my ability to make a living within my profession. They also funded my initial and continuing education with their donations (session fees). As a result, I set my fees according to my educational investments and my need to support myself and my purpose. The transpersonal perspective I've always operated under is that— whatever my purpose is here on earth, if it is supposed to sustain its existence, people will support it with financial prosperity in the long term. Otherwise, it doesn't deserve to exist or I belong doing something else that others are willing to support.

Because all relationships involve the sharing of each other's energy, the hypnotherapist's definition of the professional therapeutic relationship is an important variable. As a result, the hypnotherapist must occasionally question why they are a hypnotherapist, and if there is a benefit to themselves from doing so. Is it a healthy benefit for client and therapist? Is it one that comes from a locus of spiritual commitment and strength?

I've always made sure that my purpose for being a hypnotherapist was spiritual and not personal. In other words, I'm a hypnotherapist because it is a spiritual life-purpose and not because I need for people to like me or tell me I'm a good person. There's no personal need involved. As a result, my spiritual purpose for being in the work, which is between me and my creator, obviously serves as a primary source of strength.

Most clients are only in hypnotherapy for two or three sessions, and relationship variables are therefore rarely a factor, however, in multi-session hypnotherapy, it is more important to be attentive to the client's definition of the relationship with the hypnotherapist. Is the client attracted to the hypnotherapist? How does the client define a close relationship? How does this relationship compare to other close relationships from the past? It may be that the hypnotherapist is the only person that the client has felt comfortable enough to open up to. It is important to sometimes try to imagine what position we hold in the client's life through good listening or observation skills. Sometimes, clarification of views is necessary for hypnotherapy to proceed to the next most beneficial step.

Ways to keep the rules clear

a) Always charge fees when seeing the general public. As a general rule, never publicly discount fees or give free sessions. This not only cheapens the profession, but also puts the client in a role he or she may feel uncomfortable with. Clients feel most comfortable coming to pay for professional therapy and they do not want to make and manage a friendship; such would be the case in letting the client off the hook when the client expects to pay.

If a client prefers a friendship, it is often very taxing on the therapist; this client-type can easily grow dependent, although this is less likely in hypnotherapy as it is in other more long-term therapies. If the private practice operates under a sliding scale (a lower rate for lower income people), it is best for the hypnotherapist to define the professional exchange rules at the first session. Most clients are there to pay for services and love to have a professionally-based friendship that does not leave the confidentiality of the office. In other words, they can leave their problems with the hypnotherapist...they paid for this service.

b) Never spend personal time with clients. The American Psychological Association has a recommended two years before initiating a personal relationship with a current or past client. This keeps clarity in the professional relationship for both parties, and it also makes it easier for the client to be able to return for therapy in the future. If a client sees a hypnotherapist's personal side, he or she may not be able to reengage in the former professional relationship.

c) Do light structure work with friends and family. If the new student of hypnotherapy works with friends or family, it is probably best to do light structure work only (suggestive therapy, teach self-hypnosis, etc.), unless we are using a friend of family member for a research project (past life exploration, etc.), at which time it is best that both parties agree to such before commencing the session. Keep in mind that deeper character defining goals, such as with age regression, can sometimes alter a personal relationship. It may become more of a therapeutic relationship, shifting the roles of both parties.

Most hypnotherapists need time off. Friends that have become clients are no fun! The concept of *fun* for anyone working in a helping profession is a *must*, if the practitioner wants to sustain a healthy attitude while working within a field that involves transforming problems. Friends allow for an equal exchange of ideas and problems, rather than problems being shared one-way, such as in a therapeutic relationship. In friendship, regardless of the profession of each member in the relationship—therapist or whatever, friends can speak freely.

To summarize, if new hypnotherapists use light structure work with friends and family, and the relationship has existed with an air of helpfulness on the part the hypnotherapist, even before becoming a hypnotherapist, it may be an ideal situation with which to practice skills. I practiced with select friends and family for several months, before charging fees, when I was much younger and trying to get my feet wet; however, I find this approach less popular and know many new hypnotherapists who started practicing with a professional exchange the day that they received certification in the art.

Hypnotherapy vs. Counseling or Psychotherapy

I believe in the approach taught by Dave Elman in the 1950s, which is that hypnotherapy is most effective changing one problem at a time. Individuals who have a multiplicity of problems should seek other forms of treatment. From time to time, we may find that some clients are grasping for a diagnosis for themselves and have a very long list of problems that they need to discuss in talk-therapy. For these individuals, working together with other professionals in the community is a good idea. This approach not only benefits the client, but it also benefits the various therapists on a referral list that each hypnotherapist should put together for various purposes. On the list may be two or three of each practitioner: chiropractors, massage therapists, medical doctors, naturopaths, psychiatrists, psychologists, counselors, and some support groups (A.A., survivors of incest, etc.), and a few hot lines. I like to keep this ditto sheet handy for when it is needed.

Prosperity is increased through the process of referring and reciprocation. I remember an intuit who was an associate hypnotherapist that advised me in my early years of practice, "For every client you refer, you will receive ten clients back." I believe this ratio is fairly accurate, but we need to select practitioners to be put on the list who approve of our field of practice. I have found it best to make visits to professionals in my community to feel them out, before considering referrals. On a higher level, everybody has a place and a purpose in the grand scheme of things.

Even the United States Federal Government (Department of Labor) recognizes this in the Dictionary of Occupational Titles (D.O.T.), under "hypnotherapist" which is listed as number 079.157-010:

"Hypnotherapist induces hypnotic state in client to increase motivation or alter behavior patterns. Prepares client to enter hypnotic state by explaining how hypnosis works and what client will experience. Tests subject to determine degrees of physical and emotional suggestibility. Induces hypnotic state in client using individualized methods and techniques of hypnosis based on interpretation of test results and analysis of client's problem. May train client in self-hypnosis conditioning."

Transpersonal Hypnotherapy-A Divine Relationship

The relationship between client and transpersonal hypnotherapist is often seen as a divine relationship. In other words, each client that comes through the door is there by way of a higher will from the creator, or higher-power forces. It is a relationship that has personal growth and spiritual purposes for both parties.

Another spiritual concept that occurs within this relationship is that each individual gets what is of the highest value at the time the session transpires, regardless of the conscious therapeutic goals. For example, I have seen cases where some individuals gave up after the first session, because they weren't ready to delve that deeply into themselves at that time in their lives. I've also seen some clients, the minority, that didn't get the result that they entered into hypnotherapy for. In these cases, I simply served as a "stepping stone" for the client and his or her unique path through time, providing him or her with an opening for looking into him or herself, not a solution to the problem.

Conversely, I discovered how I was the final healer in the chain of therapists, when other therapists were stepping stones. In other words, some clients that occasionally came in to see me for hypnotherapy claimed that they had gone to another therapist earlier and weren't "ready for that," or prepared to confront a major issue at that time in their lives. As a result, the client dropped out of therapy. Sometime later, the client ended up in my office ready to confront it again, which made the other therapist a stepping stone and me the solution worker, or the final healer for that issue.

~

"To each and every action, there is an equal and/or opposite reaction"

Isaac Newton

~

We all love being the solution or the final healer of the condition, if possible. That's what both client and therapist strive for in the majority of sessions. Provided that the highest intention for each includes a healing or transformation, fortunately, that's exactly what transpires in most cases. Hypnotherapy is the most powerful medium for human change. Change and transformation will rapidly transpire, if all of the following variables for success exist.

A Recipe for Success:

1) The client both consciously and unconsciously wants to change
2) The highest intention of the hypnotherapist is transformation
3) There is good rapport between client and hypnotherapist
4) The hypnotherapist uses creativity and intuition in selecting tools that fit the client's goals
5) The higher power wills the desired change as foreseen at that time.

Now, whether we are a new student of hypnotherapy or a seasoned veteran, we can move forward into getting some profound results with the concepts we have learned. Getting changes through hypnosis, the most powerful and highest spiritual state in the world, is inevitable; and it is now at our finger tips. It is important to decide how we are going to use it at this point in the learning process. Perhaps we will use these tools on ourselves, to open up more deep, spiritual meditations; or maybe we will use hypnotherapy tools in our own unique way on the general public with our personal gifts and talents, thereby lessening pain, transforming problems, facilitating people in reaching their goals, and increasing their awareness of themselves and their world. Perhaps we will be at the scene of an accident some day, and we will use our tools to slow bleeding or lessen another's pain. Perhaps we will become a greater healer in our community, or society as a whole.

Our greatest teachers, the many potential clients out there—somewhere, are waiting for us on some level in the divine plan we each play a part in. Somehow, perhaps through the collective unconscious, we will synchronistically draw the most appropriate clients to us at this time... and we may ask ourselves, "When would *now* be a good time to start the rewarding journey of practicing hypnotherapy?"

Cayce Reading 3359.1 "...spirit taketh form in mind."[17]

Afterword

There are *other resources* that would help bring this book's concepts to light that are not included within its pages. These include right and left brain hemispheric dominance tests, sensory modality dominance tests, the Holmes and Reile stress test, and more. These personality profiling work sheets help hypnotherapists determine how the client may enter into and experience a state of hypnosis, how deep the trance level is likely to be achieved, and what his or her imagery experience is likely to entail. These may be found in the training manual of the National Association of Transpersonal Hypnotherapists (NATH) or the training manual of another institute or association which uses this text for teaching purposes.

In addition, readers may want to obtain other resources that may help with achieving better results with self hypnosis, or if a hypnotherapist, more success with clients. For these purposes, the publisher offers the book, *Script Magic: A Hypnotherapist's Desk Reference*, which is also available on CD-ROM. It offers numerous scripts for use with self-hypnosis, or professional hypnotherapy sessions, which have been proven over two decades to bring results. For more information on how to order related books, view the publisher's web site or request a free copy of the NATH newsletter listed in the Afterword.

Other resources that may help the student of hypnotherapy include the following:

✔Become a "Certified Hypnotherapist:"
Are you looking for a new career that is very rewarding? The National Association of Transpersonal Hypnotherapists (NATH) makes it easy to try a new career opportunity, since most of its courses are a combination of home study and in-class participa-

tion. The in-class portion of study may be done in just 4 to 5 days at one of NATH's training locations. Current regions where the author teaches entry-level courses include Toronto, Canada, Virginia Beach, VA, and parts of North Carolina. Advanced courses are generally offered in the mountains or on the beach-front in Virginia. In addition, the NATH is currently expanding its training locations into new regions and different countries through certified trainers; and there are several other approved schools by the NATH with similar training programs, all of whom use this text. To find these schools, view the NATH web site or request a free copy the NATH "Bridge" newsletter (next page).

Already certified or practicing hypnotherapy?

✔Hypnotherapy Master Certification Program:
An in-depth study of hypnotic regression therapy, with detailed practical instruction in what Dr. Chips refers to as *transformational models*.

✔Ericksonian Hypnosis Certification:
Ericksonian hypnosis, language patterns, Satir communication models, reframing, indirect suggestion, metaphor construction, rapport, and a transpersonal look at ecological uses for influence and materialization.

✔Hypnotherapy Trainer's Training Program:
A mentorship program for teaching Dr. Chips's certification training course, with speaking outlines, practicums, and exams, leading to certification, authorization, and materials use.

✔Reiki Therapy Training: Take accelerated programs from Reiki Masters, to become certified in an ancient healing art using hands-on healing. Learn the sacred symbols and hand positions that have brought profound healing to the mind, body, and spirit for centuries. Levels I, II, and Master.

✔Past-Life/Life Between Lives Certification Program:
This program is for certified hypnotherapists who want to learn a unique form of Spiritual Regression. The approach is based on information from The Tibetan Book of the Dead, and the ground-breaking work of Joe Fisher and Joel Whitten, MD, in the book Life Between Life. NATH

✔National Association of Transpersonal Hypnotherapists:
Become a member of this prestigious professional association or attend NATH's annual convention in autumn... a place where writers, trainers, and hypnotherapists from the United States and abroad come to share their expertise. The official organization which regularly publishes the "Bridge" Newsletter.

✔NATH's resource department:
A careful selection of books and tapes which are divided up into two categories: self-help for the general public, and clinical resources for the practicing hypnotherapist.

✔Self hypnosis/stress reduction workshops:
These two to three hour workshops are taught by the author in health care, corporate, and government environments. Inquire below for the author's speaking schedule and rates for traveling to your facility.

✔American Holistic University:
A flexible distance education degree program offering advanced degrees in holistic arts, which may be obtained through a combination of in-class instruction and home study, or solely through on-line instruction.

National Association of
Transpersonal Hypnotherapists (div. AHU.LLC)
Holistictree.com
AHUonline.org

Other Books by
Transpersonal Publishing

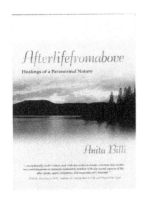
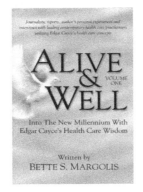
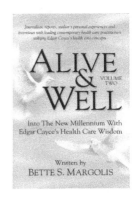

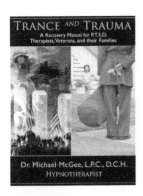
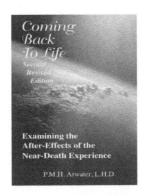
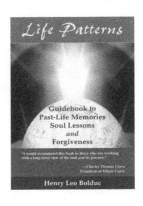

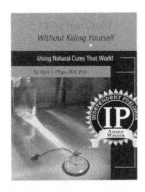
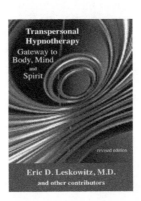
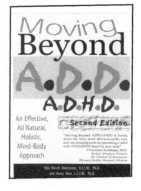

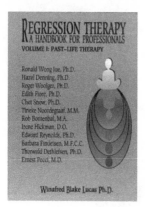

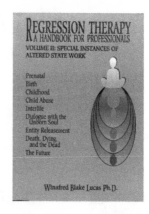

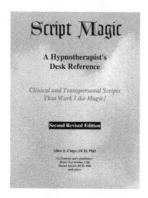

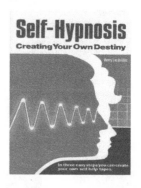

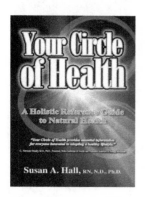

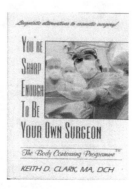

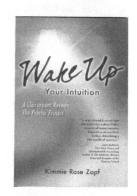

To see these and other books by the publisher, go to:
www.TranspersonalPublishing.com

GLOSSARY

Abreaction—An emotional reaction experienced by a client while under hypnosis, involving an unresolved stress within the subconscious or unconscious mind. Often a reliving or reexperiencing of negative feelings or memories under hypnosis.

Affect-bridge—An induction method by which the hypnotherapist "bridges" the client into a specific memory by way of the emotional content that the client presents during the interview in the beginning of a session.

Age Regression—Taking a client back to relive or reexperience a past memory.

Altered States of Consciousness (A.S.C.)—Those states of consciousness which deviate from a normal waking state of mind. ASC includes, but is not limited to: hypnosis, meditation, prayer, yoga, daydreaming, reiki, and biofeedback.

Alternate Realities—Areas of consciousness within the client where the imagery experienced may not be taking place on a material level, yet are significant in the fact that they reside as a reality in some dimension of either thought or matter.

Amnesia/Hypnotic—The inability of a client to recall experiences which occurred during a hypnosis session. This may be suggested to occur during hypnosis or occur spontaneously.

Animal Magnetism—*(Syn. Magnetism)* A term developed by Mesmer that described a theoretical energetic liquid in the body that responds to magnets and the stars. When out of balance, it causes illness.

Associated—A client experiences a memory, or imagery, from within the event (seeing through his/her own eyes). This effect occurs within deeper trance levels.

Association—The process by where one idea or behavior automatically triggers another behavior or idea. The effect of stimulus-response.

Attitude—A state of mind resulting from a collection of values and beliefs, which changes from day to day or moment to moment.

Auditory Sensory Modality—The sensory channel involving the perception of hearing.

Auto-hypnosis—*(Syn. Self Hypnosis);* A process by which one induces hypnosis in oneself.

Autosuggestion—A suggestion which one gives themselves during the process of self-hypnosis.

Beliefs—Value generalizations about one's world which are based in one's experiences.

Brain—The physical aspect of thought. A neural matter which science documents correlating to bodily functions and intellectual activity.

Brain Waves—As measured by the electroencephalograph, levels of consciousness or brain activity denoted by Beta, Alpha, Theta, and Delta.

Catalepsy—A condition suggested in hypnosis involving a loss of voluntary movement and increased rigidity in parts of or all of the body.

Catharsis—*(Greek Syn. Purification);* A process which may occur in hypnotic regression in which there is a discharge of suppressed emotions and intellectual concepts, leading to a purification in consciousness.

Client Interview—*(Syn. Pre-Talk);* The time period immediately before the induction of hypnosis where rapport and expectation are established during the analysis of a client's problem.

Compound Suggestion—*(Syn. Fractionation);* A deepening technique often used with resistant clients whereby the client enters and exits hypnosis repetitively.

Compulsion—An unconscious motivation or urge to behave in an impulsive fashion.

Conscious Mind—The portion of the mind which senses environmental input, and with the subconscious and unconscious information provided internally, makes decisions and judgments about specific concepts in the external environment.

Convincer—An imagination test successfully given by a hypnotherapist to a client for verifying to the client his or her hypnotic susceptibility.

Counter Suggestion—A hypnotic suggestion that is given to remedy, or counteract, problematic unconscious suggestions that exist within an individual's subconscious mind.

Critical Faculty—*(Syn. Conscious Mind);* The part of consciousness that rationalizes information which is being perceived from the environment.

Deepening Techniques—Methods used to deepen the level of hypnosis.

Dehypnotization—Procedures used for awakening a client from hypnosis.

Deletion—A filter of perception using a process of selectivity whereby people pay attention to certain aspects of their experience while deleting others from awareness.

Delusion—A false belief about things which are real, whereby hypnotized clients perceive them differently than they appear; experienced as hypnotic hallucination.

Desensitization—An advanced method of hypnotherapy involving memory repetition by which the client becomes emotionally neutral about a specific subject matter to which he or she was overly sensitized.

Dissociation—A perceptual variable, generally while experiencing a memory, whereby the client experiences a level of detachment from the memory; also a natural effect from being dissociated, or detached, from the immediate environment during induction. This in no way has any relationship to psychological dissociation.

Distortion—The universal perceptual process of distorting sensory input from the environment.

Ego—The portion of consciousness referred to as the conscious mind.

Electroencephalogram—A graphing devise used for measuring brain waves (Beta, Alpha, Theta, and Delta) thereby detecting various depth levels in consciousness.

Emotion—An internal feeling classified as part of the kinesthetic sensory modality.

Fractionation—*(Syn. Compound Suggestion);* A deepening technique whereby the client is deepened and awakened from trance repetitively; used to confuse the conscious mind of an over analytical client.

Generalization—The universal perceptual process of grouping or categorizing sensory input, in order to create meaning.

Gustatory Sensory Modality—The sensory channel involving the perception of taste.

Habit—A repetitive, unconscious behavior consistently triggered by specific stimuli within the internal and external environment.

Hallucination—A subjective, distorted perception that exists while in hypnosis which has no objective verifiability.

Heterohypnosis—The process by which a hypnotherapist puts a client under hypnosis.

Hypersuggestibility—A condition whereby a hypnotized individual is in such a deep, profound state of hypnosis that he or she experiences hypnotic suggestions immediately and almost involuntarily.

Hypnoanesthesia—A method involving techniques which cause one to become insensitive to pain stimuli.

Hypnoanalysis—A method of questioning used by a hypnotherapist to determine causative factors behind specific problems.

Hypnogogic State—An altered state of consciousness which is experienced by individuals as they cross into and out of normal sleep, or while they are lethargic.

Hypnoidal State—Typical hypnotic states of consciousness that are universally experienced while an individual is in alpha brain waves, such as daydreaming, watching television, and highway driving.

Hypnosis—Derived from the Greek word, "sleep." A particular altered state of consciousness brought about in an individual by the use of a combination of relaxation, concentration, expectation, and suggestion.

Hypnosleep—A state of mind which often begins with hypnosis and turns into a hypersuggestible state of sleep. It is detected by the behavior changes which occur as a result of suggestions given to an individual while they are in the sleep state.

Hypnotherapy—The process of using hypnosis to affect one's behavior.

Hypnotic Diet—A diet that a hypnotherapist suggests to a client for the purpose of motivating a client toward behaviors that are consistent with the goal of weight loss, weight gain, or eating modifications.

Ideomotor Response—Involuntary or unconscious activity under hypnosis experienced as a form of movement or muscular activity.

Imprint—As in Adlerian theory, the time period from birth through age eight when an individual's personality is permanently imprinted with his or her experiences, which later result in unconscious motivations.

Imagery—An internal experience involving images that occur within a person's "mind's eye" and use some or all of the five sensory modalities.

Imaginability—*(Syn. Suggestibility)*; A procedure for testing one's ability to imagine ideas to an extent that he or she will start to experience suggestions as a physical and/or mental reality.

Induction—The process of inducing hypnosis in oneself or in others .

Key—A programmed stimulus-response whereby a post-hypnotic suggestion will trigger a desired state of hypnosis.

Kinesthetic Sensory Modality—The sensory channel involving tactile sensations and feelings or emotions.

Memory—Subconscious and unconscious imagery which represents the concept of the past within one's mind.

Mesmerism—A state of hypnosis coined by the French Academy of Science to describe the healing methods of Antoine Mesmer.

Mind—The nonphysical, or metaphysical, aspect of thought.

Modeling—The act of replicating the behavior characteristics of another person.

Motivations—Inner forces within an individual which are derived from experiential ideas about specific subject matters. These ideas stimulate an individual to feel compelled toward change.

Multidimensional Self—The perceptual process within an individual which utilizes imagery for dissociation into past memories, present realities, and future potentialities during both normal and altered consciousness.

Neurolinguistic Programming (NLP)—The study of language, and other means of communication, which stimulate specific neural pathways resulting in internal experiences, or images, and affecting behavior. A reperceptual therapy.

Olfactory Sensory Modality—The sensory channel involving the perception of smell.

Operator—*(Syn hypnotist/hypnotherapist);* An individual which has the role of putting oneself or another individual under hypnosis.

Phobia—A strong fear reaction stimulated by specific subject matters or experiences.

Post Hypnotic Suggestion—Suggestions given to an individual under hypnosis to be carried out sometime after awakening.

Pre-Talk—*(Syn. Client Interview);* The time period immediately before the induction of hypnosis where rapport and expectation are established with the analysis of a client's problem.

Projection—The process of creatively imagining oneself in the future.

Psychophysical Induction—The most common hypnotic induction method by which both physical and psychological suggestions are given to relax an individual both mentally and physically.

Psychosomatic—The process by which physical ailments are caused by one's psyche, or mind.

Rapid Eye Movement (REM)—A repetitive horizontal movement of the eyes brought about in an individual while either in a state of hypnosis or sleep.

Rapid Induction—*(Syn. Instantaneous Induction);* A quick hypnotic induction method by which a hypnotherapist hypnotized or rehypnotizes a client.

Rapport—A state experienced by two individuals, due to a deep level of trust, empathy, and understanding.

Reframe—The process of reperceiving a subject matter with the intent of facilitating change.

Regression—The process of assisting a client in remembering information from his or her past, while in a state of hypnosis.

Repetition Compulsion—*(Syn. Patterns);* A theory created by Freud stating that an individual will repeat problems through various scenarios in the present that have been created or learned in the past, until he or she breaks the cycle.

Revivification—*(Syn. reliving);* An experience in which a hypnotized client experienced being associated within a memory while under hypnosis and thereby relives much of its content.

Secondary Gain—A positive reward which individuals gain consciously or unconsciously from maintaining a problematic condition.

Selective Awareness—*(Syn. Concentration);* The act of paying undivided attention to a specific subject matter.

Self-hypnosis—*(Syn. Auto-Hypnosis);* The process by which one puts themselves under hypnosis.

Sensory Modalities—The five senses of the human body, which are used to perceive both internal and external events.

Somnambulism—A deep sleep-like state of hypnosis in which the client is hypersuggestible. This state is commonly referred to as the deepest level of hypnosis.

Suggestibility—*(Syn. Imaginability);* A measure of one's capability to experience ideas described by another individual, through the use of imagination; one's ability to follow suggestions and undergo hypnosis.

Suggestion—A stimulus which implants an idea in another person's mind and automatically initiates alterations of his or her mental processes and behavior.

Subconscious Mind—An aspect of mind which provides internal representations of an individuals internal and external world by the universal process of projecting and reflecting with imagery based representations.

Subject—A person desiring to undergo hypnosis with specific motivations or expectations for doing so.

Superconscious Mind—The part of the mind that is connected to non-physical existence and spiritual experiences, including the collective unconscious and the akashic records.

Susceptibility—Research on various hypnotized subjects which proves that different populations and personality types are more susceptible to a state of hypnosis than others.

Time Distortion—A phenomenon experienced under hypnosis whereby the client overestimates or underestimates the time that he or she has been under hypnosis.

Time Line—A reference of time which is used to facilitate hypnotic age regression.

Unconscious Mind—The part of the mind which holds amnesiac memories—those that are not readily available to the conscious mind in a normal waking state of consciousness.
Visual Sensory Modality—The sensory channel involving the perception of sight or seeing.

Waking Hypnosis—A term often used by Milton Erickson to describe how human beings enter into subtle hypnotic states on a regular basis.

Will Power—A conscious effort by an individual to select certain subconscious images, while avoiding others, in order to control his or her own behavior.

Footnotes

1
C.T. Tart, *Altered States of Consciousness*, ed. N.E Zinberg (New York: Free Press, 1977), pp. 1-6

2 A.M. Ludwig, *Altered States of Consciousness*, (Arch Gen Psychiat 15, 1966), pp. 225-34

3 Errol R. Korn, M.D. and Karen Johnson, M.A., *Visualization: The uses of Imagery in the Health Professions*, (Homewood, IL, Dow Jones-Irwin, 1983) pp. 39-53

4 F.A. Pattie, *Mesmer's Medical Dissertation and its Debt to Mead's De Imperio*, ed. Solis ac Lunae. (J. Med. Allied Science, 1956), 11:275

5 Milton Erickson, *My Voice Will Go With You: The Teaching Tales of Milton H. Erickson*, ed. Sydney Rosen, M.D., (New York-London, W.W. Norton and Company, 1982) pp. 80-81

6Jesus Christ, *The New English Bible*, ed. Rev.-Dr. C.H. Dodd (Oxford University Press; Cambridge University Press, 1962) Matthew 9:22, p. 16

7 Errol R. Korn, M.D. and Karen Johnson, M.A., *Visualization: The Uses of Imagery in the Health Professions*, (Homewood, IL, Dow Jones-Irwin, 1983) p. 61

8 C. Goldfarb, J. Driesen, and D. Cole, *Psychophysiologic Aspects of Malignancy*, (Am J Psychiatry 123, June 1967) p. 1546

9 Masud Ansari, *Modern Hypnosis: Theory and Practice*, (Washington, DC, Mas-Press, 1991) p. 31

10 Dave Elman, *Hypnotherapy*, (Glendale, CA, Westwood Publishing Co.) pp. 95-117

11 Wilda B. Tanner, *Mystical Magical Marvelous World of Dreams*, (Tahlequah, OK-Sparrow Hawk Press), p. 16

12 J.H. Conn, *Is Hypnosis Really Dangerous?*, (International Journal of Clinical and Experimental Hypnosis, 1972) 20: pp. 60-79

13 J.G. Watkins, *Anti-Social Compulsions Induced Under Hypnotic Trance*, (Journal of Abnormal Social Psychology, 1947), 42:256

14Edgar Cayce, *The Complete Edgar Cayce Readings on CD-ROM*, (Virginia Beach, The Edgar Cayce Foundation, 1994), portions of readings 3742.2 and 900.31

15 C.G. Jung, *Memories, Dreams, Reflections*, ed. Anela Jaffe, (New York-Vintage Books), pp.137-138

16 C.G. Jung, *Memories, Dreams, Reflections*, ed. Anela Jaffe, (New York-Vintage Books), p. 138.

17 Edgar Cayce, *The Complete Edgar Cayce Readings on CD-ROM*, (Virginia Beach, The Edgar Cayce Foundation, 1994), portions of reading 3359.1

Index

Symbols

no entries

A

B

W

X

no entries

Y

no entries

Z

no entries

"Imagination is more important than knowledge."

Albert Einstein